Trends in Wound Care, Volume IV

edited by
Keith F Cutting

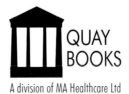

QUAY
BOOKS

A division of MA Healthcare Ltd

Quay Books Division, MA Healthcare Limited, St Jude's Church,
Dulwich Road, Herne Hill, London SE24 0PB

British Library Cataloguing-in-Publication Data
A catalogue record is available for this book

ISBN 1 85642 309 3

Printed by Gutenberg Press Ltd, Gudja Road, Parxien, Malta PLA 19

Contents

List of contributors

Elizabeth Ayello is Professor of Nursing, Division of Nursing, New York University, New York, USA

Anne Ballard Wilson is Tissue Viability Nurse, Queen Margaret Hospital, Dunfermline, Fife

Margaret Broadbent is Clinical Nurse Specialist, Central Sydney Area Health Service, Sydney, Australia

Naomi Burbridge is Tissue Viability Nurse Specialist, Islington Primary Care Trust (also covering Camden PCT and Camden and Islington Mental Health Care Trust), London

Gayle Burr is Senior Academic, Retired, Faculty of Nursing, University of Sydney, Australia

Hellen Casey is Clinical Nurse Specialist, Central Sydney Area Health Service, Sydney, Australia

Marianne Cummins is Clinical Nurse Consultant in Older Persons Acute Care, Division of Medicine, John Hunter Hospital, Newcastle, New South Wales

Keith F Cutting is Principal Lecturer, Buckinghamshire Chilterns University College, Shalfont St Giles, Buckinghamshire, and Director of Health Directions, Chorleywood, Hertfordshire

Caroline Dowsett is Nurse Consultant in Tissue Viability, Newham Primary Care NHS Trust, London

Helen Hollinworth is Senior Teaching Practitioner, Suffolk College, Ipswich

Jane James is Tissue Viability Nurse, West Wales General Hospital, Carmarthenshire NHS Trust

Sarah Kiernan is Tissue Viability Nurse Consultant, Islington Primary Care Trust (also covering Camden PCT and Camden and Islington Mental Health Care Trust), London

Diane L Krasner is Staff Development Nurse, VNA Home Health Services, York, Pennsylvania, USA

Ellie Lindsay is Independent Specialist Practitioner and Associate Lecturer, Thames Valley University, London, and Visiting Fellow, Queensland University of Technology

Miles E Maylor is Senior Lecturer in Tissue Viability, School of Care Sciences, University of Glamorgan, Pontypridd, Mid-Galmorgan

Marie McMullen is Tissue Viability Nurse Specialist, Epsom and St Helier University NHS Trust, Epsom Hospital, York House, Epsom

Amelia Merriman is Clinical Nurse Consultant, Aged Care Psychiatry, Northern Sydney Health/Hope Healthcare North, Sydney, Australia

Rachael Osborne is Junior Sister, Suffolk Coastal Primary Care Trust

Catherine Sharp is Wound Care/Infection Control Consultant, University of New South Wales, Sydney, Australia

Noleen Smith is Third-Year Medical Student, Guy's, King's and St Thomas' Hospital, London

David Tillman is Senior Clinical Lecturer, Dermatology Section, Faculty of Medicine, University of Glasgow

Patricia Tyler is District Nursing Sister, Suffolk Coastal Primary Care Trust

Kathryn Vowden is Nurse Consultant, Bradford Teaching Hospitals NHS Foundation Trust, and Lecturer, School of Health Studies, University of Bradford, Bradford

Foreword

Once again, our colleagues in wound care across the pond have taken a leadership role internationally by producing this fourth body of work in the *Trends in Wound Care* series in association with the *British Journal of Nursing*. Kudos to all the contributors to *Trends in Wound Care, Volume IV* and to editor Keith Cutting, who has so skillfully directed this book!

The first three volumes in the *Trends in Wound Care* series (2001, 2003, 2004) deal primarily with the nuts and bolts of wound care — aetiologies, assessment techniques, prevention strategies, the evidence-base for interventions and other foundational aspects of wound care. This fourth volume shifts the focus to the cutting edge of advanced wound care and wound research.

The 12 chapters address a variety of clinical issues and research challenges, from assessment to advanced adjunctive therapies. Common issues that patients face emerge as themes over and over again, such as pain, impact on quality of life and the challenge of co-adherence. All of the studies presented, be they descriptive, qualitative or quantitative, shed light on the complexity of advanced wound care.

Time and again the astute reader will be stuck by the multivariate nature of the phenomena related to wound care and the challenge of designing research that will not only yield statistically significant results, but also clinically significant results. The research included in this volume serves as a model for designing meaningful research studies for wound care.

This book is a gift to the world of wound care. It is certain to open readers' eyes and hearts to see and feel the needs of people with wounds quite differently. Again, sincere thanks to the contributors and editor for giving us new eyes and new insights to help address the challenges of advanced wound care.

'The real voyage of discovery
Consists not in seeking new landscapes
But in having new eyes.' Marcel Proust

Diane L Krasner
PhD RN CWCN CWS FAAN
October 2005

Chapter 1

Signs and symptoms of hypothetical wound assessment by nurses

Miles E Maylor

This chapter reports from a study in which tissue viability nurses, MSc student nurse practitioners and postregistration nurses on a wound management module ($n = 61$) ranked signs and symptoms of wound healing, stasis and deterioration relative to their supposed importance. The top ranked sign for a healing wound was 'size' (reduction), for a static wound was 'no' (change) and for a deteriorating wound was 'increase' (pain). This was a convenience sample, and caution is indicated in generalizing results. However, there were statistically significant differences between assessors in the number of words they used (ANOVA; $P < 0.001$), and in the words they used for different wound phases (χ^2; $P < 0.001$). The study supports the view that there are some words used in common by different respondents in specific wound phases. However, a previous study raised questions about what people actually mean when they use a particular word (Maylor, 2003).

The word 'wound' represents the sum of many parts. At the broadest level, there is not much dispute as to what constitutes a wound, but wounds are subject to dynamic processes of change. Furthermore, wound assessment involves both objects (such as amount of slough) and processes (such as change in slough over time).

This chapter reports findings of a study into the words and concepts that underpin wound assessment. It illustrates the conclusion that wound assessment is intrinsically difficult to capture in words, and also raises the intriguing possibility that there are different descriptors and thought processes involved in different phases of the 'life' of a wound. It could be argued that inter-rater reliability will only increase when account is taken of the trajectory of the wound, i.e. either towards healing or deterioration. Further, there is evidence that static wounds are mainly judged by the absence of signs and symptoms, perhaps based on an expected mental image of a wound. Therefore, wound assessment might need a different approach from its current documentation and methods of measurement to allow phase-related information to be used more coherently.

Literature review

A literature search was undertaken in August 2004 to identify studies that investigated terminology used by wound assessors. Databases included CINAHL, Journals@Ovid, EMBASE, PubMed and MEDLINE. Key words used singly, with derivatives and in combination, were: 'wound', 'ulcer', 'assessment', 'method', 'preference', 'learning style', 'terminology', 'word' and 'consensus'.

One article reported a study of problems inherent in using words in wound assessment, and called into question the assumption of current expert consensus on the use of such words (Maylor, 2003). Another article discussed the problem of a lack of defined terms in researching wound care, and a call was made to agree useful datasets for information (Fletcher, 2003).

No other articles were found to address the issue of terminological preferences of assessors specifically. One article dealt with clinical decision making with reference to documentation of wounds (McGuiness and Axford, 1997). The authors pointed out that clinicians use spatial and visual clues, but are expected to document this via linguistic interpretation. Also, they concluded that photographic methods of recording could potentially reduce differences in perception between novices and experts, although this was a convenience sample ($n = 49$ postgraduate student nurses) and did not reach statistical significance. Further, they assumed that expert agreement was the standard to judge by, even though the least experienced nurses tended to be more accurate in their identification of wound features than those with more experience.

The findings of another study indicated that there are problems in assuming that there is consensus on the use of common words in wound assessment (Maylor, 2003). Further, where consensus does not exist on the meaning of an assessment criterion (such as the size of a wound), respondents would use additional words to justify their own description. A consequence of this is that wound assessment could get even more complex, rather than simpler.

Aims

This study is the second part of a sequence (see Maylor, 2003) aimed to identify words that could be applied to specific wound phases. It also aimed to provide information for a new method of assessment that would take into account the personality of the wound assessor and his/her information-processing preferences.

Sample and method

A convenience sample of 61 respondents included postregistration students ($n = 34$) on a diploma-level wound management course, and MSc student nurse practitioners ($n = 11$) attending a lecture on wound care; 16 tissue viability nurses were chosen because they were all employed directly and full time in the field of tissue viability. They were asked personally and by email if they would participate.

Anonymized views were collected using a single A4 proforma with three columns: column A for healing; column B for stasis; and column C for deterioration. The rubric asked participants to state in as few words as possible what they thought were signs and symptoms for these categories of wound. After listing these, they should rank the three signs or symptoms in each of the columns that they considered to be most important (A = most important, B = second most important, C = third most important). Ethical approval to use anonymous data gleaned alongside teaching sessions had been given by the university research committee, and all the participants willingly agreed to take part.

A database (Microsoft Excel) was used to separate phrases into words that would appear in columns associated with the context of healing, stasis or deterioration. This enabled them to be analyzed in separate categories of wound (e.g. healing, static or deteriorating). All of the words were given a unique identification number, and the data were exported for analysis into Statistical Package for Social Scientists (SPSS) version 11.0.

Results

The top 20 most frequent signs and symptoms that respondents say they look for in a healing wound are shown in *Table 1.1*. The columns A, B, and C indicate that respondents ranked these as the first (A), second (B), and third (C) most important sign to them of healing. Of a total of 138 different words suggested for all three phases of wounds, only 78 (56.5%) of them were used in the healing category.

Table 1.1: Top 20 words mentioned as indicators of important signs and symptoms of healing in wounds

Words used	Rank A healing	Rank B healing	Rank C healing	Total
Size	5	50	4	59
Granulation	29	11	5	45
Wound	8	14	9	31
Reduce	8	11	9	28
Epithelialization	2	10	5	17
Decrease	2	3	11	16
Tissue	10	4	2	16
Exudate	1	5	9	15
No*	1	3	7	11
Less	3	2	6	11
Pain	2	1	8	11
Inflammation	4	5	1	10
Healthy	6	1	2	9
Bed	5	3	0	8
Red	5	0	1	6
Clean	2	1	2	5
Presence	1	3	1	5
Good	3	2	0	5
Swelling	2	1	1	4
Blood supply	2	2	0	4

* 'No' was self-evidently used in conjunction with other words, e.g. no slough

The top 20 most frequent signs and symptoms that respondents say they look for in a static wound are shown in *Table 1.2*. Of 138 different words suggested for all three phases of wounds, 93 (67.4%) were applied to stasis.

Table 1.2: Top 20 words mentioned as indicators of stasis in wounds

Words used	Rank A stasis	Rank B stasis	Rank C stasis	Total
No*	29	29	37	95
Change	15	14	14	43
Wound	16	9	3	28
Reduce	11	8	8	27
Size	10	6	5	21
Granulation	6	5	6	17
Exudate	3	7	4	14
Bed	7	3	0	10
Pain	4	3	3	10
Slough	1	4	4	9
Oedema	3	2	2	7
Tissue	4	2	1	7
Continuous	3	2	1	6
Signs	2	2	2	6
Unhealthy	4	1	0	5
Dimension	0	0	5	5
Epithelialization	0	4	1	5
Inflammation	4	1	0	5
Presence	1	0	3	4
Remains	3	1	0	4

* 'No' was self-evidently used in conjunction with other words, e.g. no slough

The top 20 most frequent words that respondents mention for a deteriorating wound are shown in *Table 1.3*. Of 138 different words suggested for all three phases of wounds, 78 (56.5%) were applied to deterioration.

Table 1.3: Top 20 words mentioned as indicators of signs and symptoms of deterioration in a wound				
Words used	**Rank A deterioration**	**Rank B deterioration**	**Rank C deterioration**	**Total**
Increase	20	17	19	56
Pain	10	8	7	25
Wound	11	3	8	22
Exudate	5	9	8	22
Infection	5	6	6	17
Slough	2	8	6	16
No*	3	5	7	15
Size	5	3	4	12
Inflammation	7	0	2	9
Tissue	2	4	1	7
Breakdown	4	2	1	7
Odour	2	3	3	8
Oedema	0	4	2	6
Deteriorate	3	1	1	5
Surrounding	2	3	0	5
Areas	3	1	1	5
Discharge	2	2	1	5
Absence	0	2	2	4
Red	3	0	1	4
Bed	3	0	1	4

* 'No' was self-evidently used in conjunction with other words, e.g. no slough

A number of respondents failed or declined to rank signs and symptoms relative to each other. Further, it appears that the lower the perceived importance of the sign or symptom (*Table 1.4*), the more people declined or refused to rank it. In other words, they might put something in a column (for healing, stasis or deterioration) but then only feel able to rank A, but not B or C; or A and B, but not C. This implies that they were increasingly uncertain about the importance of some signs and symptoms. Alternatively, they could have been asserting that only A, or A and B were important.

Table 1.4: Refusal or failure to rank signs and symptoms by number of respondents

	Unranked A	Unranked B	Unranked C	Total
Static phase	5	11	18	34
Deteriorating phase	1	4	7	12

NB. In the healing phase there was no failure to rank signs and symptoms

From a total pool of 138 possible words, an interesting pattern emerges in their suggested usage or non-usage. The first point is that healing and deterioration appear to have an axial or polar relationship, having the same proportions of numbers of words mentioned or not mentioned (*Table 1.5*). The second point is that there are more words suggested for stasis than for the other two phases. Put differently, it takes more words to express stasis than other phases. This is supported by the fact that proportionately more unique words are suggested for stasis than for healing or deterioration.

Table 1.5: Count of words suggested more than once, once only, and not used from a pool of 138

	Healing	Stasis	Deterioration
Numbers of words mentioned more than once	90 (65.2%)	87 (63.0%)	90 (65.2%)
Number of words mentioned once only	31 (22.5%)	40 (28.9%)	31 (22.5%)
Number of words not mentioned relative to each phase	59 (42.8%)	47 (34.1%)	59 (42.8%)

Discussion

In healing wounds, size is clearly important to these respondents (see *Table 1.1*). However, despite being cumulatively the most important it is largely ranked 'B', whereas granulation is mostly ranked 'A'. This could mean that people in some way understand size to be of clear importance to most respondents, but not of the first rank of importance; whereas granulation is of proportionately more importance to some respondents than it is for others. Further, as the wound goes from healing to static to deteriorating, size decreases in importance — in other words, it is mentioned less frequently.

'No' is the top mentioned word in the static phase, but of equal frequency in healing and deteriorating wounds (see *Table 1.2*). Also, the word 'change' ranks second to top in stasis, whereas it does not feature in the top 20 at all for healing, and only twice for deterioration. This could indicate that respondents predominantly classify static wounds in terms of no change. Further, 'presence' is mentioned in healing (5) and stasis (4), and 'absence' in deteriorating wounds (4). This might indicate an underlying search for confirmation of imagined features of a phase, which depends on a person's memory (McGuiness and Axford, 1997).

An introductory rubric requested that respondents use as few words as possible to note their opinions on the proforma. Nevertheless, the word 'wound' is consistently highly mentioned for all three phases. In one sense, this could be thought to be redundant or obvious — indeed it often was, as granulation could only be in the wound. However, it could also mean that people did not think of wound assessment or care simply in terms of the wound itself, hence the inclusion of the words 'margins', 'skin' and 'surrounding' tissues elsewhere. Alternatively, they just did not read the rubric.

Caution should be exercised when using statistics as the sample was opportunistic and no claims are being made that participants represent the population of wound assessors. However, for this sample (tissue viability nurses, nurse practitioner students and postregistration students on a wound course), there were differences in the total number of words used per wound phase (ANOVA (analysis of variance); $F = 12.388$, d.f. (degrees of freedom) $= 60$, $P < 0.001$). There is a trend for tissue viability nurses to use more explanation and, therefore, more words than other nurses. Further, there were differences between the words most frequently mentioned for the three phases of wound ($\chi^2 = 274.9$, d.f. $= 10$, $P < 0.001$). More research would be needed to understand or confirm these differences.

Some respondents decided, either by omission or refusal, not to rank signs and symptoms relative to importance. Two respondents were excluded from analysis for explicitly saying they could not rank any items. One of these said that all signs and symptoms were equally important. However, as rank went from A to B to C, there was a pattern of increasing omission (see *Table 1.4*) and there is an implied rank. Second, signs and symptoms associated with the static phase may be less easy to rank or to discern than in the deteriorating or healing phase of wounds (all were ranked in the latter). Self-evidently, this raises issues about the validity and reliability of signs and symptoms in different wound phases, probably implying that consensus is less easy to achieve in these phases.

To date, no literature has been found that discusses learning styles and personality types in relation to wound assessment. Everyone has their own preference in how they learn and how they express their personality (Myers and Myers, 1995; Clack et al, 2004). The Myers–Briggs Personality Type Indicator (MBTI) has been extensively validated as a means of describing how people prefer to react to information from the world (Borges and Savickas, 2002; Jessup, 2002). Although this study was not specifically designed to test the relationship between personality type or learning style, it has produced data that can be explained in relation to them. For example, in the MBTI, sensors let 'the eyes inform the mind' and intuitors are personality types who prefer to let 'the mind inform the eyes' (Miller, 1995). Sensors perceive information in terms of what they think their senses tell them. Intuitors look for possibilities, meaning and relationships from the immediate to the bigger picture (Francis and Jones, 2000; Francis and Atkins, 2001). In this study many were similar to intuitors, and others closer to being sensors. Each type can learn from and use the other's preferences if they choose. However, it is too simplistic to assume that they are speaking with total mutual comprehension.

Limitations

As mentioned above, this was a convenience sample and, as such, it is not possible to generalize the conclusions to a population. Also, the majority of respondents were interested in wound care to the extent that they were specialists in the field, or had opted to study it at diploma level. Despite there being such an interest in wound care in this sample, there were many specialties covered, and this could have biased the words they chose to reflect knowledge from their areas of work. In practice, there are many levels of interest, expertise and professions involved in wound assessment, so further study might show whether different professions or levels of involvement with wounds has any effect on the words mentioned.

The study involved using memory and active speculation about what to include as wound descriptors. This method depends on cognition, interpretation and recall, all of which could be investigated in terms of validity of words mentioned in this context (McGuiness and Axford, 1997). Similarly, some people have better memories or interpretation than others. Influences of previous wound assessment forms (WAFs) on choice of words is likely to be important, but was not researched as such. As a previous study showed (Maylor, 2003), caution should be used when assuming that the words people use in common actually mean the same to both parties. In the present study, the meaning of the words has not been further critiqued and it is likely that some respondents have understood certain words in a different sense than others. An example of possible ambiguity is the word 'inflammation' when 'infection' is meant (Edwards et al, 2002).

Conclusions

Recently the literature has presented methods of assessment that take account of outcomes and of how treatment affects the characteristics of a wound over time (Bolton et al, 2004; Browne et al, 2004; Keast et al, 2004). The 'TIME' principles describe the relationship between clinical observations and clinical outcome (Schultz et al, 2003). Clinical observations are: tissue non-viable or deficient; infection or inflammation; moisture imbalance; edge of wound non-advancing or undermined. They are designed:

> '... to help the wound care practitioner make a systematic interpretation of the observable characteristics of a wound' (Dowsett and Ayello, 2004).

Two other recent methods systematize data recording relevant to treatment effectiveness — the 'TELER' method (Browne et al, 2004) and the 'MEASURE' framework (Keast et al, 2004). However, all these methods involve practitioners choosing, justifying and interpreting their knowledge, then applying it to the method — they put in what they think is appropriate in their own terms (TELER, 2004). Boyd et al (2004), in the context of chronicity, developed a tool to identify whether a wound has factors that would predispose it to non-healing. They stress the importance of looking for signs of healing in a holistic way. Therefore, perhaps the key development in recent wound assessment methodology has been the increased importance of judging wound progress relative to time, but all methods depend on cognition and personal interpretation of signs and symptoms.

Apart from Maylor (2003), no other work has been traced that explores wound assessment in terms of the meaning of words and concepts being communicated between practitioners. This present part of a sequence of studies raises questions that could impinge on the design of WAFs and on education about wound assessment. For example, is there any point in trying to record stasis if this is difficult to express and is really judged by the absence of signs rather than the presence of distinct features of a phase?

Subsequent analysis of the words revealed that there are subjective and objective words, and some that depend on previous knowledge or cognition. Also, conceptual examination has linked the respondents' personality type (MBTI) with preferences in choice of wound assessment words. The implication of the latter is that a 'one-size fits all' WAF does not sufficiently account for differences of perception linked to the personality (or learning style) of the assessor. Further, personal 'imagination' seems to be an intrinsic part of wound assessment (perhaps calling into mind a hypothetical or 'ideal' wound — healing or otherwise). Reliability studies need to factor these matters into their analysis.

References

Bolton L, McNees P, Van Risjwijk L et al (2004) Wound healing outcomes using standardized assessment and care in clinical practice. *J Wound Ostomy Continence Nurs* **31**(2): 65–71

Borges NJ, Savickas ML (2002) Personality and medical choice: a literature review and integration. *J Career Assess* **10**(3): 362–80

Boyd G, Butcher M, Glover D, Kingsley A (2004) Prevention of non-healing wounds through the prediction of chronicity. *J Wound Care* **13**: 265–6

Browne N, Grocott P, Cowley S et al (2004) Wound care research for appropriate products (WRAP): validation of the TELER method involving users. *Int J Nurs Stud* **41**: 559–71

Clack GB, Allen J, Cooper D, Head JO (2004) Personality differences between doctors and their patients: implications for the teaching of communication skills. *Med Educ* **38**(2): 177–86

Dowsett C, Ayello E (2004) TIME principles of chronic wound bed preparation and treatment. *Br J Nurs* **13**(Suppl 15): S16–S23

Edwards LM, Moffatt CJ, Franks PJ (2002) An exploration of patients' understanding of leg ulceration. *J Wound Care* **11**: 35–9

Fletcher J (2003) Standardizing the methodology of research into chronic wounds. *Prof Nurse* **18**: 455–7

Francis LJ, Jones SH (2000) The relationship between the Myers-Briggs type indicator and the Eysenck Personality Questionnaire among adult churchgoers. *Pastoral Psychol* **48**(5): 377–86

Francis LJ, Atkins P (2001) *Exploring Matthew's Gospel: A Guide to the Gospel Readings in the Revised Common Lectionary.* Continuum International Publishing Group, Mowbray

Jessup CM (2002) Applying psychological type and 'gifts differing' to organizational change. *J Organizational Change Manage* **15**(5): 502–11

Keast DH, Bowering K, Evans AW, Mackean GL, Burrows C, D'Souza L (2004) MEASURE: a proposed assessment framework for developing best practice recommendations for wound assessment. *Wound Repair Regen* **12**(Suppl 3): S1–S17

McGuiness B, Axford R (1997) Exploring nursing knowledge by using digital photography. *Stud Health Technol Inform* **46**: 281–7

Maylor M (2003) Problems identified in gaining non-expert consensus for a hypothetical wound assessment form. *J Clin Nurs* **12**: 824–33

Miller VG (1995) Characteristics of intuitive nurses. *West J Nurs Res* **17**(3): 305–16

Myers IB, Myers PB (1995) *Gifts Differing.* Consulting Psychologists Press, Palo Alto, California

Schultz GS, Sibbald RG, Falanga V (2003) Wound bed preparation: a systematic approach to wound management. *Wound Repair Regen* **11**(2): 1–28

TELER (2004) *The TELER® Concept.* TELER Ltd, Sheffield (http://www.teler.com/teler_overview.asp#Concept) (last accessed 9 March 2005)

Chapter 2

Quality of life and leg ulceration from the patient's perspective

Anne Ballard Wilson

Chronic leg ulceration can have a profound impact on a patient's quality of life. Studies have shown that pain and general interference with normal activities of living are the major themes emerging that are often not dealt with in a consistent manner by healthcare professionals. A literature review of this subject shows that although a number of studies have been carried out on quality of life related to chronic leg ulceration, there is little evidence that these findings are being addressed in the daily management of these often complex leg ulcer patients. This chapter examines the research relating to quality of life and leg ulceration, and determines what the most important issues are from the patient's perspective, in an effort to improve the way nurses manage their care.

Chronic leg ulceration is thought to affect up to 2% of the adult population in the UK and Ireland (Callam et al, 1985, O'Brien et al, 2000) and is a condition that can have a significant impact on quality of life. Healing rates are low and there is often recurrence of the ulceration. In the author's experience the management of patients with chronic leg ulceration is often poor, with too little emphasis placed on the importance of a holistic approach to care.

Hayes (1997) asserts that the trauma, stress and loss of dignity experienced by the patient with a chronic leg ulcer is often understated. Charles (1995a) carried out a small study on patients with leg ulceration and found that healthcare professionals often do not listen to them or understand their healthcare issues. Healthcare workers also commonly assume that venous leg ulcers are not painful, and little consideration is given to assessing pain in a routine leg ulcer assessment (Krasner, 1998).

The term quality of life was first used during the 1990s in relation to healthcare issues, in an attempt to define patients' experience of their illness (Price, 1993). From a review of the literature available on this subject, it is clear that there are a number of issues that range from defining what quality of life means for the patient to studies undertaken that give us insight into the difficulties patients with chronic leg ulceration face. This chapter examines and evaluates the literature to show how nurses involved in leg ulcer management can use research information to improve the overall quality of life for patients.

A literature search was undertaken using OVID online, with searches of CINAHL, MEDLINE, Cochrane Systematic Reviews and the British Nursing Index databases. The search terms used were 'leg ulceration' and 'quality of life'. It is recognized that there may be differences in the types of symptoms perceived between different types of ulceration that could affect quality of life, but these were not examined in this review.

Defining quality of life

In 1996, the European Tissue Repair Society met to try and reach an agreement on defining quality of life for patients with chronic wounds (Price, 1996). While recognizing that it would be difficult to come to a consensus, it looked at a number of issues relating to this subject, emphasizing that the patient is the key, as only he/she can understand the significance of his/her experience. Price (1993) states that:

> '... *quality is something that we all feel we can recognize but that is notoriously difficult to define*'.

Many clinicians question the concept of quality-of-life issues as having broader implications and prefer to see it as a 'personal assessment of life satisfaction' (Price and Harding, 1996). Barrett and Teare (2000) argue that quality of life can be subjective as it is defined by the individual's expectation of the disease and his/her ability to cope with it.

Fallowfield (1990) set out four core domains in an attempt to analyze quality of life. These domains were concerned with the effects of disease on various areas of a person's daily life and included psychological, social, occupational and physical aspects. Bowling (1991) described quality of life as a concept that represented an individual's response to the physical, mental and social effects of illness on daily living. These represent two examples of earlier generic quality-of-life tools that do not attempt to measure issues specifically related to living with a chronic wound. Today, two generic tools used frequently in research are the Nottingham Health Profile (NHP; Hunt et al, 1986) and the Short Form 36 (SF-36; Ware and Sherbourne, 1992). These will be discussed in more depth as part of the review of studies looking at leg ulceration and quality of life. Price (1996) recognized that no matter which tool is used, it must reflect the problems of the patient group under investigation.

Quality-of-life studies

Price (1996) carried out a study of 55 patients using the SF-36 (*Table 2.1*), a tool developed in the USA. She found statistical significance in seven of the eight subscales, finding that patients with leg ulcers experienced more pain, less vitality and more restriction in their physical and social functioning when compared with the UK normal, which was based on the healthy population aged 70–74 years.

Table 2.1: Domains of two generic assessment tools

Short Form-36	Nottingham Health Profile
Physical functioning	Energy
Social functioning	Pain
Physical role limitation	Emotional reactions
Emotional role limitation	Sleep
Pain	Social isolation
Vitality	Physical mobility
General health perception	
Mental health	

From Hunt et al (1986); Ware and Sherbourne (1992)

In a much larger study of 758 patients using the NHP (see *Table 2.1*), Franks and Moffatt (1998) found that leg ulceration had a major impact on patients' health-related quality of life, with the main features again being pain, mobility and energy. They also found that there was a greater impact on the quality of life of younger male patients, with men scoring higher than women in the domains of bodily pain, sleep and social isolation. The main reasons cited for this were related to the method of analysis and the age/sex mix of patients. It is argued that there must be an adjustment made for the age of the patient, as there was a higher impact on perceived quality of life in younger patients within the study.

In a large study of 125 patients using the NHP, Lindholm et al (1993) found that males showed remarkably elevated scores, especially in the areas of pain, emotional reactions, social isolation and physical restrictions. Another interesting finding in this study was that the duration of the ulcer did not appear to influence quality of life, suggesting that patients use adaptive or coping mechanisms to deal with long-term ulceration.

Smith et al (2000) conducted a prospective study of 98 patients using the SF-36 in combination with an ulcer-specific questionnaire that demonstrated good reliability. They argue that it is preferable to use both a generic and a specific measure of quality-of-life tool when assessing a condition. It is suggested that use of a generic tool alone may miss important influences on the quality of life of patients with leg ulcers; for example the effects that treatments such as compression bandaging might have. *Table 2.2* lists some of the disease-specific issues related to leg ulcer care posed to the participants of this study.

Table 2.2: Disease-specific issues related to leg ulcer care

Appearance of ulcer

Leg swelling

Smell/discharge from ulcer

Ulcer interferes with cooking/cleaning/shopping

Dressing a problem: bulkiness/appearance/clothes

From Smith et al (2000)

In a study of 65 patients, Charles (2004) found that there was a significant improvement in quality of life when a combination of good wound management and effective compression therapy were used. Although a generic tool was used in this study (the SF-36), other data analyzed included an investigation of the differences between whose ulcers did and did not heal, as well as gender and age of the patient.

Smith et al (2000) demonstrated high levels of validity in correlating the scores obtained from the 'divisions' of the ulcer questionnaire with the domains of the SF-36. The questionnaire was shown to be 'responsive', meaning that its final score decreased appropriately as the ulcer healed.

Hamer and Roe (1994) carried out a study into patients' perceptions of their leg ulcer disease and the impact it had on their quality of life. Data were obtained from a total of 88 patients with leg ulcers and 77 without. The study discusses preliminary results related to findings. When asked 'what is the worst thing about your leg ulcer?', over a third of the respondents stated pain, with just under a third stating restriction of mobility.

Several of the research studies found in the literature related to the use of phenomenology, first conceived at the beginning of the 20th century by Husserl (1962), a German philosopher. Its aim is to focus on an individual's interpretation of his/her experience. Beck (1994) suggests that:

'... phenomenology affords nursing a new way to interpret the nature of consciousness and of an individual's involvement in the world'.

Using a descriptive, phenomenological approach, Krasner (1998) carried out research into 14 patients with painful venous ulcers. The main themes developing were frustration, interference with work, significant life changes and finding satisfaction in new activities. She also discussed other studies that challenge the assumptions made that venous leg ulcers are not painful, showing that up to 78% of participants interviewed experienced pain. These findings are reinforced by Charles (1995a), who also used a phenomenological approach in her small study involving four patients. She found that pain was the most overwhelming experience for all patients.

In a study of 62 patients, Phillips et al (1994) found that 65% reported severe pain related to their ulcer. These studies are important as they highlight the need to assess pain more thoroughly as part of the overall leg ulcer assessment.

Loftus (2000) undertook a longitudinal quality-of-life study that compared four-layer bandaging systems with superficial venous surgery for treatment of venous leg ulcers. This study used the EuroQol quality-of-life questionnaire alongside a disease-specific questionnaire designed by the author. Although this was a relatively small study with only 15 patients, no other studies to date have compared the effects of different treatments on quality of life in these patients. Therefore, the results, which again show that pain was a major issue, are interesting. Both groups showed an improvement in quality of life, with a more marked improvement in the bandage group — this was thought to be related to these patients receiving regular visits from a nurse who may have advised them and assisted them with pain control. Loftus argues that:

'When initiating treatment, reducing the pain experienced should be a major consideration.'

The idea of a longitudinal approach to research in chronic leg ulceration is an appropriate one, as phenomena can develop over time that affect the attitude, belief and behaviour of the sufferer (Parahoo, 1997). For example, an improvement in leg ulcer pain levels over time may mean that a patient can return to normal activities, which in turn could affect mood and behaviour, and ultimately healing of the ulcer.

A study undertaken by Douglas (2001) looked at eight patients with leg ulceration of over 1 year's duration. Using a qualitative approach, five major categories developed, which included physical and psychological effects. It was seen that these appeared to be heavily influenced by the relationship between the patient and the healthcare professional. Patients and carers often felt that they had little knowledge or control of their treatment, demonstrating a need for nurses to improve their communication with patients.

Moffatt (2004) discusses patient concordance in her article, which examines issues related to the interaction between patients and practitioners. She argues that we must develop our skills in reflective professional practice and look at our attitudes and behaviour, which may exacerbate patients' suffering and contribute to poor concordance with treatment.

In an interesting commentary as an adjunct to Krasner's (1998) study, Dr Gary Sibbald discusses the importance of qualitative information and how it helps us develop a holistic approach to patient management. He goes on to discuss the need for reflecting on our practice, and argues that this will improve our effectiveness as healthcare providers. *Table 2.3* lists quality-of-life issues raised within this

Table 2.3: How quality-of-life issues can be improved for patients

Our holistic approach: did we involve or network with others in the interdisciplinary team?

Did we spend 3–5 minutes listening to the patient without interrupting?

What measures did we take to create a caring context and a caring relationship with the patient?

How did we ensure that the '3Cs' (consistent, connected, concernful) of care were attended to? (the follow-up)

How did we support the coping mechanisms (work, recreation, general activities such as bathing) of the patient? (life changes)

Extract by Gary Sibbald from Krasner (1998)

study, which are suggested for use when assessing patients with leg ulcers.

Bland (1996) raises a subject that is often discussed, that some patients with leg ulcers do not want them to heal because they want to continue their contact with nurses. She also discusses the 'knitting needle syndrome', a phrase used by nurses to describe what patients do to prevent ulcers from healing, such as 'poking a knitting needle inside the bandage to scratch at the ulcer'. Her small study of nine patients was carried out in New Zealand, and was mainly concerned with how patients coped with their leg ulceration. She states that as many patients must live with their ulcers for many years, the real challenge must be to make life as normal as possible for them while continuing to promote wound healing.

An extensive literature search by Anand et al (2003) looked at health-related quality-of-life tools for venous-ulcerated patients. They suggest that there are several disease-specific tools available for measuring quality of life in these patients. It is argued that one of the most difficult tasks is to choose a tool for assessment that has an acceptable level of validity, reliability and responsiveness. Their recommendation of a tool for addressing these issues is the Freiburger Lebensqualitaet Assessment Questionnaire (FLAQ), developed by Augustin et al (1997). It consists of 83 items that cover a wide range of issues related to patients with leg ulcers. The author claims that it takes an average of 21 minutes to complete the questionnaire; however, it is published in German so it would be interesting to see how well it would translate into English. Another consideration would be how many elderly patients suffering from leg ulceration would be able to complete such an indepth questionnaire.

Case studies of patients with leg ulcers

On reviewing the literature, there were a number of articles relating the 'stories' or experiences of patients with leg ulceration. It would be easy to dismiss some of these case study articles as they have individual perspectives, but case studies play an essential role in helping nurses understand the issues that patients face when coping with their leg ulcer. One particular article, written by a patient, was extremely moving and brought home some of the issues, such as pain and fear, that he experienced (Woodall, 1996):

'Sometimes, I feel there is so much wrong with me that I shall end up by being too expensive for the practice.'

'My wife will wake me but the worst part of the day follows, when I go

along to the bathroom to shave. I am afraid to put my feet to the ground.'

Charles (1995b) describes some of the experiences of patients with leg ulcers:

'Pain was terrible...God almighty, the pain was terrific...it was unrelenting.'

Mobility was also an issue:

'I couldn't walk about...I packed up driving...I was on crutches...I couldn't take the kids swimming...I didn't go out.'

In a case study by Flurrie (2001), the effects that pain had on one particular patient were examined. She found that the nursing documentation did not allow for adequate evaluation of pain, demonstrating to her that a true holistic approach to care for that patient was not achievable.

Another case study by Taylor (1999) includes a patient's diary and demonstrates how compression bandaging improved that patient's quality of life. Her description of 'jumping', 'tingling' and 'burning' in her leg ulcer gradually tails off as it begins to improve and ultimately heal.

Conclusion

There are many quality-of-life issues to be considered in the care of patients with chronic leg ulceration. From reviewing the literature, it is clear that a truly holistic approach must be taken to manage these patients effectively. Scherwitz et al (1997) discuss the 'placebo effect', arguing that if a patient thinks that he/she is being treated effectively, the outcome can be improved. Nurses must work with patients and help them to face the issues within their daily lives that they perceive to be problems, rather than just assuming what their problems are. Only by listening to patients and allowing time for them to relate their experiences will their management be improved. Anderson (2000) discusses the time constraints that nurses face today and argues that, despite this, attention must be made to promoting quality of life in patients with leg ulcers.

One of the main issues highlighted in almost every quality-of-life study carried out on patients with leg ulcers is that of pain. This appears to be poorly addressed in many areas. There is currently no research evidence on the availability of specific pain assessment tools for leg ulcers. It is interesting to note that the Scottish Intercollegiate Guidelines Network (SIGN) guidelines did not address the issue of pain in venous ulceration, seeing it as being 'complex and outwith the remit of this guideline' (SIGN, 1998). This is something that needs to be addressed in any future guideline development.

The studies discussed in this literature review are varied, with both generic- and disease-specific tools used. It is recognized that a combination of the two will lead to a better understanding of the issues affecting the patient with a leg ulcer. The FLAQ tool, as discussed by Anand et al (2003), was found to be the most appropriate disease-specific tool, but to the author's knowledge there has been no study using this tool in the UK.

Many of the studies reviewed had relatively small patient numbers; however, it is recognized that this was because of the mainly qualitative approaches used as there can be difficulties conducting larger studies of this nature. When looking at issues experienced by patients with leg ulcers, a phenomenological approach is an excellent way of exploring themes; even though patient numbers may be small, valuable information can be obtained (Krasner, 1998).

Patients with chronic leg ulceration present a huge challenge to many nurses in both primary and secondary care. Flanagan (2001), in her study looking at community nurses, carers and patients' perceptions of factors affecting leg ulcer recurrence and management of services, showed that health promotion was ineffective, and leg ulcer after-care services fragmented. She discusses the need for a strategy to support 'healing behaviour', which will potentially reduce recurrence and improve quality of life. Ruane-Morris (1995) recognizes the concept of 'patients for life', and argues that care should be 'long term and across all settings'.

Nurses must work with their colleagues in the future to develop a consistent and caring approach to managing patients with chronic leg ulceration. If assessment of quality of life became a routine part of the patient's assessment, it would vastly improve our understanding of the patient's needs.

The author gratefully acknowledges the support given by Alison Coull in the preparation of this chapter.

References

Anand SC, Dean C, Nettleton R, Praburaj DV (2003) Health-related quality of life tools for venous ulcerated patients. *Br J Nurs* **12:** 48–59

Anderson (2000) Quality of life and leg ulcers: will NHS reform address patient need? *Br J Nurs* **9**: 830–40

Augustin M, Dieterle W, Zschocke I et al (1997) Development and validation of a disease-specific questionnaire on the quality of life of patients with chronic venous insufficiency. *Vasa* **26**(4): 291–301

Barrett C, Teare JA (2000) Quality of life in leg ulcer assessment: patients' coping mechanisms. *Br J Community Nurs* **5**: 530–40

Beck CT (1994) Phenomenology: its use in nursing research. *Int J Nurs Stud* **31**: 499–510

Bland M (1996) Coping with leg ulcers. *Nurs NZ* **2**(3): 113–14

Bowling A (1991) *Measuring Health.* Open University Press, Buckingham

Callam MJ, Ruckley CV, Harper DR, Dale JJ (1985) Chronic ulceration of the leg: extent of the problem and provision of care. *Br Med J* **290**: 1855–6

Charles H (2004) Does leg ulcer treatment improve patients' quality of life? *J Wound Care* **13**(6): 209–313

Charles H (1995a) The impact of leg ulcers on patients' quality of life. *Prof Nurse* **10**: 571–4

Charles H (1995b) Living with a leg ulcer. *J Community Nurs* **July:** 22–4

Douglas V (2001) Living with a chronic leg ulcer: an insight into patients' experiences and feelings. *J Wound Care* **10**: 355–60

Fallowfield L (1990) *The Quality of Life: The Missing Dimension in Health Care.* Souvenir, London

Flanagan M (2001) Community nurses', home carers' and patients' perceptions of factors affecting venous leg ulcer recurrence and management of services. *J Nurs Manag* **9**: 153–9

Flurrie KL (2001) Care study: the effect of pain on a patient with leg ulcers. *Br J Nurs* **10**: 868–78

Franks PJ, Moffatt CJ (1998) Who suffers most from leg ulceration? *J Wound Care* **7**: 383–5

Hamer C, Roe BH (1994) Patients' perceptions of chronic leg ulcers. *J Wound Care* **3**: 99–101

Hayes M (1997) Quality of life in patients with chronic leg ulceration. *J Wound Care* **6**: 348–9

Hunt SM, McEwan J, McKenna SP (1986) *Measuring Health Status.* Croom Helm, London

Husserl E (1962) *Ideas: General Introduction to Pure Phenomenology.* Collier, New York

Krasner D (1998) Painful venous ulcers: themes and stories about their impact on quality of life. *Ostomy Wound Manage* **44**(9): 38–49

Lindholm C, Bjellerup M, Christensen OB, Zederfeld B (1993) Quality of life in chronic leg ulcer patients. *Acta Derm Venereol (Stockh)* **73**: 440–3

Loftus S (2000) A longitudinal, quality-of-life study comparing four-layer bandaging and superficial venous surgery for the treatment of venous leg ulcers. *J Tissue Viabil* **11**(1): 14–19

Moffatt CJ, (2004) Perspectives on concordance in leg ulcer management. *J Wound Care* **13**(6): 243–8

O'Brien JF, Grace PA, Burke PE, (2000) Prevalence and aetiology of leg ulcers in Ireland. *Int J Med Sci* **169:** 110–12

Parahoo K (1997) *Nursing Research, Principles, Process and Issues.* Macmillan Press, London

Phillips T, Stanton B, Provan A, Lew R (1994) A study of the impact of leg ulcers on quality of life: financial, social and psychologic implications. *J Am Acad Dermatol* **31:** 49–53

Price P (1993) Defining quality of life. *J Wound Care* **2:** 304–6

Price P (1996) Quality of life meeting. *J Wound Care* **5:** 103

Price P, Harding K (1996) Measuring health-related quality of life in patients with chronic leg ulcers. *Wounds* **8**(3): 91–4

Ruane-Morris M (1995) Supporting patients with healed leg ulcers. *Prof Nurse* **10:** 765–9

Scherwitz LW, Rowntree R, Delevitt P (1997) Wound caring is more than wound care: the provider as a partner. *Ostomy Wound Manage* **43**(9): 42–56

Scottish Intercollegiate Guidelines Network (1998) *The Care of Patients with Chronic Leg Ulcers.* SIGN/Royal College of Physicians, Edinburgh

Smith JJ, Guest MG, Roger M, Greenhalgh MA, Chir M, Davies A (2000) Measuring the quality of life in patients with venous ulcers. *J Vasc Surg* **31:** 642–93

Taylor A (1999) Life with venous leg ulcers: the story of one patient. *Community Nurse* **5**(6): 39–40

Ware JJ, Sherbourne CD (1992) The MOS 36-item short-form health survey (SF-36). I. Conceptual framework and item selection. *Medical Care* **30:** 473-83

Woodall RD (1996) Living with leg ulcers: a patient's personal experience. *Nurs Stand* **10**(45): 52

Chapter 3

The relationship between pain and leg ulcers: a critical review

Marie McMullen

Leg ulceration may have a profound impact on the individual: in some cases activities of living become subservient to the degree of pain experienced. Pain control, which is viewed as a key function in health care, appears marginalized in leg ulcer management. Pain can be intense, bringing psychological implications for the patient. Knowledge deficiency in practitioners' management of venous and arterial leg ulcers was identified in the literature. This may lead to unnecessary pain caused by inappropriate dressings, misdiagnosis or poor technique in the use of compression therepy. A holistic approach to the patient using evidence-based, standardized practice may improve the patient's experience.

A leg ulcer may be defined as a wound occurring on the lower leg that takes more than 6 weeks to heal (Dale et al, 1983). It may be arterial, venous (Figure 3.1) or diabetic in origin. Pain is inherently difficult to define owing to its subjective nature and differential pain thresholds across different individuals (Tyrer, 1992). Arterial ulcers have been acknowledged as painful, but recent studies have indicated that venous ulcers can also produce pain (Moffatt, 1998; Dealey, 2001). Pain in leg ulcers is cited in the literature as a symptom of infection and arterial disease and, in some cases, is ignored by practitioners (Charles, 2002).

Leg ulceration has been shown to be a profoundly complex issue, rarely understood by practitioners (Hofman, 1997). From the patient's perspective, leg ulceration may eclipse other conditions judged by the practitioner as more onerous, such as diabetes (Hyde et al, 1999). The patient's activities may become subservient to the leg ulcer and the degree of pain experienced. Pain

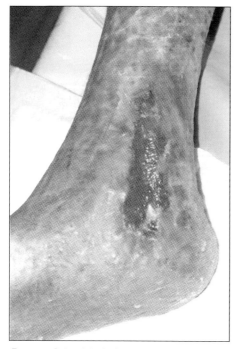

Figure 3.1: Medial venous ulcer that caused excruciating pain to the patient

control, which is seen as a key function in health care, appears marginalized in leg ulcer management (Dealey, 2001).

The impact of painful leg ulcers on quality-of-life issues are frequently misunderstood by carers (Hollinworth, 2000), and inappropriate management can lead to litigation (Culley, 2000). Dimond (2003) argues that failure to assess and manage the patient appropriately could be interpreted as a breach of the Human Rights Act 1998. In addition, recent government initiatives, such as *Making a Difference* (Department of Health (DoH), 1999a), alongside *Guidelines for Practice* (Nursing and Midwifery Council (NMC), 1996) emphasize higher levels of accountability in providing quality care. Despite this, there appears to be an inconsistency between research findings and clinical practice that warrants further scrutiny.

This chapter looks at the literature in relation to pain and leg ulcers, and highlights the importance of pain control in leg ulcer management.

Literature search strategy

The key words 'leg ulcers' and 'pain' were searched using a year range of 1994–2004. Medline, Cinahl and the British Nursing Index (BNI) produced 100 research studies. Cinahl and Medline databases yielded a collective total of 83 research studies; the BNI yielded 17. Hand searches were made of recent issues of *Journal of Wound Care*, *Journal of Tissue Viability* and conference proceedings. National and international literature was deployed to broaden the research perspective.

Owing to the plethora of studies retrieved, the search was confined to literature focusing on the impact of pain in patients with leg ulcers and how it is managed by practitioners.

Literature review

One of the emergent themes was the profound impact that a leg ulcer can have on the life of the individual (Ebbeskog and Ekman, 2001). In many patients it became the dominant factor in health from their perspective. Ebbeskog and Ekman (2001) conducted a phenomenological–hermeneutic study into elderly persons' experience of living with a venous leg ulcer. Fifteen patients between the ages of 74–89 years attending a primary healthcare clinic in Stockholm, Sweden, were selected. Audio-taped interviews using open-ended questions were the main method of data collection. The results indicated that life activities were subordinate to the ulcer and the level of pain experienced. The findings emphasized the importance of seeing life with an ulcer from the patient's perspective.

The main methodological strength of this type of research is that it can produce a wealth of rich data, and may provide an opportunity for the interviewer to seek clarification if needed (Ogier, 1998). Conversely, Burnard (1991) highlights the difficulty in the interpretation of such material, for example in deciding which part of the analysis to include or exclude, as each person's world view is potentially valid.

Similar research by Hyde et al (1999) was conducted, producing a descriptive study using indepth interviews on 12 women with venous leg ulcers aged between 70–93 years. Participants were treated by the Sydney home nursing team, Australia. The results indicated two emerging themes: the patients' endeavours in gaining control over pain, leakage, smell and skin and limb integrity; and dealing with lifestyle consequences of impaired mobility and chronic leg ulceration.

In common with the previous research study, interviewees may be able to express views more easily verbally rather than in writing, and therefore provide more flexibility for the researcher and interviewee (Ogier, 1998). Pre-existing conditions such as arthritis, common in older people, may also contribute to pain and immobility (Schofield, 2003). It is not clear from these studies as to whether the interviewees' pain was caused by ulcers or by other factors, such as arthritis.

The problem of patients living with considerable and sometimes constant pain emerged as another primary theme in the literature (Hofman, 1997). The evidence suggested that pain was perceived as an accepted part of having an ulcer, and not seen as something that could be reduced or more appropriately managed (Nemeth et al, 2003). The complexity of pain, with its accompanying emotional and psychological impact, was rarely addressed. This becomes evident in the following three studies that attempt to examine the prevalence of pain in patients with leg ulcers.

Hofman (1997) conducted a 6-month prospective study using a convenience sampling method. One hundred and forty patients with venous leg ulcers from two centres (Oxford, UK and Malmo, Sweden) were studied. A semistructured questionnaire and a visual analogue scale (VAS) were employed. The results of the study indicated that pain in leg ulcer patients was inadequately controlled; 69% of patients cited that pain was the worst thing about having a leg ulcer.

A methodological strength of the study is that two methods were used (Crookes and Davies, 1998), thereby providing more robust evidence. A weakness of the VAS in this study is that it may be inaccurate in patients with poor eyesight. It can also lead to social desirability bias as the patients may give the response they perceive the practitioner would prefer them to give (Cormack, 1996). The ability to generalize this study's finding may be limited owing to the sampling method. Polit and Hungler (1999) argue that convenience sampling is rarely representative of the target population, and therefore has a potential for bias. Additionally, this study focuses on patients attending clinics, when it is well documented that most patients receive care at home (Royal College of Nursing (RCN) Institute and University of Manchester, 1998). Practice implications may be limited as the study was conducted in two centres with different health systems, producing an incongruency in outcomes.

Nemeth et al (2003) conducted a non-probability longitudinal study over three seasons (autumn, winter and spring). Selected from a Canadian community leg ulcer service, 250 patients with pure and mixed aetiology venous leg ulcers were deployed. A pain assessment scale, the numerical rating scale (NRS) and a structured questionnaire were the main methods of data collection. The study concluded that most patients had severe pain and considered the ulcer the worst problem despite having other significant medical problems. For younger working people, the ulcer was correlated with job loss, time off from work and financial difficulties. The methodological strength of this study was that longitudinal studies allow for changes in trends and phenomena over time, thereby presenting a realistic long-term view (Crookes and Davies, 1998). Conversely, Polit and Hungler (1999) point out that the time or season that the data is collected can influence people's emotions or behaviour, thereby affecting study variables. The fact that the study concluded in spring rather than winter may produce a response bias.

Administering the same questionnaire and VAS three times may have given rise to response bias. Crookes and Davies (1998) argue that respondents' familiarity with the tools can alter the outcome; however, if conducted some months apart, as in this study, it may not be such an issue (Cormack, 1996). The chief methodological weakness in this study is the use of convenience sampling. DeVaus (1986) argues that this method of sampling can only be extrapolated to the local or study population, and not to the population at large. As mentioned earlier, it is unlikely to be representative of the population, as not everyone had an equal chance of selection. Additionally, the findings of a Canadian study may not be extrapolated to a UK setting.

Charles (2002) conducted a longitudinal repeated measure design into the characteristics of venous leg ulcer pain. Sixty-five patients were randomized to one of three treatment groups over 12 weeks. All patients received short-stretch bandaging. Data were collected using the McGill Pain Questionnaire (Melzack, 1975) and a VAS at 2-weekly intervals. The study demonstrated that 71% of all patients reported moderate to severe pain associated with the ulcer at entrance; following treatment this reduced to 10% at exit, with a 65% healing rate.

Randomization with a repeated measure design is considered a powerful method of data collection. The same group of individuals are used throughout and act as their own control, therefore extraneous variables are reduced (Cormack, 1996). A methodological limitation of the study is the use of psychometric scales, which are susceptible to response bias, social desirability bias and acquiescence, especially among older people (Polit and Hungler, 1999). The results may also be flawed because of the 'placebo' effect of having frequent expert attention, which in itself may produce pain relief and healing (Hollinworth, 2000). Clinical implications of this study may be limited as candidates had ulcers for 3–4 months only, and patients with immobility or insulin-dependent diabetes were excluded. Most leg ulcers are chronic in nature, many with accompanying immobility problems or other complications such as diabetes (RCN Institute and University of Manchester, 1998). It could be argued, therefore, that the candidates recruited for this study were not typical.

A third theme that emerged from the literature was a knowledge deficiency in practitioners in the management of leg ulcers (Lorimer et al, 2003). This may lead to unnecessary pain and discomfort in patients, caused by inappropriate dressings, misdiagnosis, lack of empathy or poor technique in the use of compression bandaging (Hollinworth, 2000).

Two studies (Dealey, 2001; Lorimer et al, 2003) examined nursing practice in the management of leg ulceration: one in the community and one in the acute setting. Lorimer et al (2003) conducted an audit of the nursing documentation of 66 patients with venous leg ulcers receiving care from a Canadian nursing agency. Using non-probability sampling, the study aimed to determine the congruency of community care using a checklist reflecting three critically appraised practice guidelines: the RCN Institute and University of Manchester (1998), the Scottish Intercollegiate Guidelines Network (1998) and the Clinical Resource Efficiency Support Team (1998).

The results of the study concluded that only 15% of clients (10/66) were assessed for pain, and that a number of care practices were incongruent with recommended guidelines. The study highlighted the importance of a standardized approach to care. The primary methodological strength of this study is that it may be an effective method in providing a baseline for future improvements (Donabedian, 1988).

Mann (1996) suggests, however, that effective changes in practice will only occur if there is a detailed action plan stating exactly who, when, what and how changes are to be made. A methodological weakness is that this study (Lorimer et al, 2003) relies heavily on accurate documentation, and lack of anonymity may lead to a response bias (Polit and Hungler, 1999). The findings may be transferred to the UK as the guidelines were UK in origin. One of the methodological limitations of non-probability sampling in this article, as supported by Crookes and Davies (1998), is its potential for bias.

Dealey (2001) conducted a case study methodology on six patients with leg ulcers in an acute hospital, to determine the level of nursing knowledge. Method triangulation using nursing knowledge questionnaire, participant observation and patient interviews was the main method of data collection. The results indicated a knowledge deficit in nurses caring for a leg ulcer patient: many had received little training resulting in less than optimum care. Four out of the six patients identified pain as a major factor. However, it is not clear from the study whether the nurses acted on this information. The primary methodological strength of the study is that triangulation is perceived as a robust method in establishing validity and credibility (Carr, 1994). A methodological limitation is that the results will have local significance and cannot be extrapolated into the wider setting (Ogier, 1998).

While both studies set out to examine nursing practice in patients with leg ulcers, improvements may be limited unless a multidisciplinary approach is established (Vowden and Vowden, 1998). Ideally, nurses need to work in collaboration with the vascular team, dietitians, tissue viability specialists and so on, to provide holistic care for the patient by sharing expertise.

Finally, the availability of quality-of-life tools for accurate assessment and documentation of patients with leg ulcers was identified in the literature. Franks et al (2003) conducted a longitudinal study on 118 patients with chronic leg ulceration receiving treatment in the community setting using the SF-36 questionnaire to assess quality of life. The questionnaire was deployed at the start of the study and after 12 weeks. The study concluded that there was a significant reduction of pain experienced after the ulcer was healed, and that the SF-36 was a reliable indicator of quality-of-life issues. The main methodological strength is that it used a repeated method design that controlled for subject variation during the period between the two measurements (Polit and Hungler, 1999). A methodological weakness is that familiarity with the questionnaire can compromise outcome, and subjects may experience the 'halo effect' when behaviour of the respondents is altered owing to being the focus of a study (Polit and Hungler, 1999).

The results of the questionnaire may have been determined by other factors, such as treatment used, care standards or pain management — variables which are not mentioned in this study (Franks et al, 2003). The use of this questionnaire may, however, serve to improve practice outcomes by identifying and acting upon quality-of-life issues at an earlier stage.

Pain control

Pain in leg ulcer management is frequently seen as inevitable by patients and nursing staff; however, there are strategies that may be employed to help eradicate or reduce pain (Hyde et al, 1999; Nemeth et al, 2003). A reduction in leg ulcer pain may be achieved by a pain assessment so that the most effective analgesia may be prescribed; for example patients that complain of neuropathic pain will need a different analgesia from those who experience pain caused by vascular disease (Briggs et al, 2002). A multidisciplinary approach to pain relief, such as the involvement of a pain specialist nurse, is recommended (Briggs et al, 2002). Non-pharmacological strategies such as diversional or relaxation interventions may be employed (Melzack and Wall, 1988).

A standardized, evidence-based approach to leg ulcer management and the understanding by practitioners that venous as well as arterial ulcers can be painful may improve the patient's experience (Hollinworth, 2002). The use of non-stick dressings, which may prevent trauma at dressing change (e.g. hydrofibres or hydrogels), instead of gauze or paraffin tulle, can minimize trauma at dressing change (European Wound Management Association, 2002).

Clinical practice implications

Recent government initiatives have placed increased importance on evidence-based practice (DoH, 1999a,b). While there appears to be a concerted effort to move away from ritualistic, task-oriented practice towards holistic, evidence-based nursing, this chapter suggests that there is need for further improvement in leg ulcer management. Staff training and education in standardized, evidenced-based practice is needed. Staff should not be expected to perform skills, such as for compression therapy, without evidence of competency. A holistic assessment of the patient incorporating quality-of-life issues and pain assessment may serve to improve the patient's experience. A multidisciplinary approach by collaborating with the vascular surgeon, tissue viability nurse, pain specialist nurse or GP is recommended for best practice (RCN Institute and University of Manchester, 1998).

Application of the reviewed research findings may serve to empower the nurse's role of advocate, reduce the financial and emotional cost of leg ulceration, and reduce the number of complaints and litigation.

Conclusion

This critical review of the literature has shown that leg ulceration is a profoundly complex issue rarely understood by practitioners. From the patient's perspective, life activities may become subservient to the leg ulcer and the degree of pain experienced. Leg ulceration may totally eclipse other medical conditions judged by the practitioner as more onerous. Quality-of-life issues, such as embarrassing odour or leakage from the ulcer, assume greater importance than those conditions perceived more onerous by practitioners (Hyde et al, 1999). Pain can be intense, bringing psychological implications for the patient.

The review has further demonstrated that it is a fallacy to assume that only arterial ulcers are painful. A further find of the review is a knowledge deficit in the assessment and management of leg ulcers by some practitioners in the community as well as in the acute setting. Pain control, which is seen as a key function in health care, appears marginalized in leg ulcer management. More qualitative research is needed regarding the patient's experiences of leg ulceration. Further research in the management of chronic painful wounds is recommended.

References

Briggs M, Torra I, Bou JE (2002) Pain at wound dressing changes: a guide to management. In: *European Wound Management Association Position Document. Pain at Wound Dressing Changes.* Medical Education Partnership, London

Burnard P (1991) A method of analyzing interview transcripts in qualitative research. *Nurse Educ Today* **11:** 461–6

Carr LT (1994) The strengths and weaknesses of quantitative and qualitative research: what methods for nursing? *J Adv Nurs* **20:** 716–21

Charles H (2002) Venous leg ulcer pain and its characteristics. *J Tissue Viabil* **12**(4): 154–8

Clinical Resource Efficiency Support Team (1998) *Guidelines for the Prevention and Management of Pressure Sores.* CREST Secretariat, Belfast

Cormack DFS (1996) *The Research Process in Nursing.* 3rd edn. Blackwell Scientific, Oxford.

Crookes P, Davies S (1998) *Research in Practice.* Ballière Tindall, London

Culley F (2000) Legal and professional issues in tissue viability revisited. *Wound Care Society Educational Leaflet* **7**(1)

Dale J, Callam M, Ruckley C, Harper D, Berrey P (1983) Chronic ulcers of the leg: a study of prevalence in a Scottish community. *Health Bull* **41:** 310–4

Dealey C (2001) Care study methodology in tissue viability part 2: a study to determine the levels of knowledge of nurses providing care for patients with leg ulcers in an acute hospital setting. *J Tissue Viabil* **11**(1): 28–34

Department of Health (1999a) *Making a Difference: Strengthening the Nursing, Midwifery and Health Visiting Contribution to Health and Health Care.* The Stationery Office, London

Department of Health (1999b) *The New NHS: Modern, Dependable.* The Stationery Office, London

DeVaus DA (1986) *Surveys in Social Research.* Allen & Unwin, London

Dimond B (2003) Pressure ulcers and litigation. *Nurs Times* **99**(5): 61–3

Donabedian A (1988) The assessment of technology and quality. *Int J Technol Assess Health Care* **4:** 487–96

Ebbeskog B, Ekman SL (2001) Elderly persons' experience of living with venous leg ulcers: living in a dialectal relationship between freedom and imprisonment. *Scand J Caring Sci* **15**(3): 235–43

European Wound Management Association (2002) *Pain at Wound Dressing Changes: The Use of Diversion.* European Wound Management Association, London

Franks P, McCullagh L, Moffatt C (2003) Assessing quality of life in patients with chronic leg ulceration. *Ostomy Wound Manage* **49**(2): 26–32

Hollinworth H (2000) Pain and wound care. *Wound Care Society Educational Leaflet* **7**(2)

Hollinworth H (2002) How to alleviate pain at wound dressing changes. *Nurs Times* **98**(44): 51–2

Hofman D (1997) Pain in venous ulcers. *J Wound Care* **6**(5): 222–24

Hyde C, Ward B, Horsfall J, Winder G (1999) Older women's experience of living with chronic leg ulceration. *Int J Nurs Pract* **5**(4): 189–98

Lorimer K, Harrison M, Graham I, Friedberg E, Davies B (2003) Venous leg ulcer care: how evidence-based is nursing practice? *J Wound Ostomy Continence Nurs* **30**(3): 132–42

Mann T (1996) *Clinical Audit in the NHS. Using Clinical Audit in the NHS: A Position Statement.* Department of Health, London

Melzack R (1975) The McGill Pain Questionnaire: major properties and scoring methods. *Pain* **1**(3): 277–99

Melzack R, Wall PD (1988) *The Challenge of Pain.* 2nd edn. Penguin Books, London

Moffatt C (1998) Issues in the assessment of leg ulceration. *J Wound Care* **7**(9): 469–73

Nemeth KA, Harrison MB, Graham ID, Burke S (2003) Pain in pure and mixed aetiology venous leg ulcers: a three-phase point prevalence study. *J Wound Care* **12**(9): 336–40

Nursing and Midwifery Council (1996) *Guidelines for Practice.* NMC, London

Ogier M (1998) *Reading Research.* Ballière Tindall, London

Polit D, Hungler B (1999) *Nursing Research: Principles and Methods.* 6th edn. Lippincott Williams & Wilkins, Philadelphia

Royal College of Nursing Institute and University of Manchester (1998) *Clinical Practice Guidelines: The Management of Patients with Venous Leg Ulcers.* RCN, London

Schofield P (2003) Pain assessment: how far have we come in listening to our patients? *Prof Nurse* **18**(5): 276–9

Scottish Intercollegiate Guidelines Network (1998) *The Care of Patients with Chronic Leg Ulcers.* SIGN, Edinburgh

Tyrer S (1992) *Psychology, Psychiatry and Chronic Pain.* Butterworth-Heinmann, Oxford

Vowden K, Vowden P (1998) Venous leg ulcer assessment part 2: assessment. *Prof Nurse* **13**(9): 633–8

Chapter 4

The wearing of compression hosiery for leg problems other than leg ulcers

Patricia Tyler, Helen Hollinworth, Rachael Osborne

Many people have leg problems other than ulceration. Practitioners from one primary care trust in Suffolk considered nursing assessment of these patients and the fitting of prescribed compression hosiery where appropriate as a health promotion initiative. However, ongoing assessment adds to heavy clinical demands on community practitioners. Engaging with people to take greater responsibility for their health, and recognition that practice should be underpinned by credible evidence, provided the backdrop to a two-staged retrospective audit. Results are based on the nursing records of 101 patients wearing prescribed compression hosiery other than for previous venous ulceration. It was concluded that following an initial detailed holistic assessment, including ankle brachial pressure index, those patients who meet identified characteristics can be empowered to return for reassessment only if there is a change in their health status or skin changes to their legs. An information leaflet is considered critical to this strategy.

Leg ulcer care has undergone many developments since dedicated clinics were established as part of the Charing Cross and Riverside Leg Ulcer Project during 1988 (Dowsett, 2004). Subsequent research has demonstrated improved healing rates and more ulcer-free weeks with patients treated at community clinics, rather than at home (Morrell et al, 1998). In Suffolk, many district nursing teams responded by setting up leg clinics during the late 1990s. As well as treating leg ulcers, these clinics offered assessment of people with leg problems other than ulceration. This was seen as a health-promotion initiative and it was hoped that many possible future ulcers would be avoided. People could self-refer, or be referred by GPs and other health professionals. Many of these people were fitted with appropriate compression hosiery, and high satisfaction rates were reported in an informal local survey. There was a huge latent demand for this service, far greater than had been anticipated.

In June 2001, Suffolk district nurses formed a Leg Care Forum to share good practice and discuss practice issues. One topic discussed was the problem of ongoing assessments for the now significant number of patients wearing compression hosiery. It was agreed that all patients with a past history of leg ulceration must be regularly assessed in line with the Royal College of Nursing (RCN, 1998) guidelines. The guidelines state that frequency of reassessment can be determined by local protocols, even though Simon et al (1994) recommend 3-monthly Doppler reassessments for patients with leg ulceration because of advancing arterial disease. However, this research has subsequently been criticized because it had no control group, the technique for ankle brachial pressure index (ABPI) measurement was out of date, there was a risk of referral bias and healing time was not taken into account (Pankhurst, 2004).

The issue highlighted by the Forum related to people wearing compression hosiery for reasons other than previous venous ulceration.

A literature search was carried out using Cinahl and the British Nursing Index for the year range 1992–2002. In addition, a hand search was undertaken of the Journal of Wound Care. The key words used were 'compression hosiery', 'intact skin', 'varicose veins', 'oedema' and 'prevention of deep vein thrombosis' (other than that relating to surgery). It found no studies relating to assessment/reassessment of people wearing compression hosiery for aching legs or to prevent varicose veins or deep vein thrombosis development. It was not considered appropriate, therefore, to produce a local protocol about the frequency of reassessment for these people without some evidence to underpin safe practice. A steering group of nurses from across Suffolk was formed in May 2002.

Methods

The initial plan, through an informal audit, was to identify 'high-risk' patients who would require ongoing assessment because of their high risk of having a decreasing ABPI (indicative of advancing arterial disease). However, we were advised that our investigations should be carried out in a more structured way in order for the results to have validity. With no relevant research as a starting point, we sought the advice of a vascular surgeon based in Suffolk. He confirmed that a list of the characteristics that led to people wearing compression hosiery being considered 'high-risk' had not been formulated, and suggested the way forward was to carry out a retrospective audit to help identify high-risk patients. Funding to carry out the audit was sought without success, but the project continued with the support of lecturers at the higher education institution in Suffolk.

Data collection and analysis

Stage one

In early 2003, a detailed scrutiny of nursing documentation was carried out for 128 patients from Suffolk Coastal Primary Care Trust (PCT) wearing compression hosiery for reasons other than leg ulcer prevention/management. Nursing management permission was obtained before commencement. Assessment of these patients and nursing documentation has always reflected evidence-based practice (RCN, 1998; Vowden and Vowden, 2001) and professional standards (Nursing and Midwifery Council (NMC), 2002a,b). A large quantity of data was generated, which was then analyzed and reviewed by the steering group, all of whom were practitioners skilled in the care of leg ulcer patients. Patient characteristics were based on more than 80% of the patients having that characteristic. Rather than being able to identify high-risk patients clearly, this strategy exposed the characteristics of those people wearing compression hosiery (class I or class II) for leg problems other than past or present ulceration.

Table 4.1: Characteristics of patients wearing compression hosiery (class I or class II) for leg problems other than past/present ulceration: inclusion criteria

No diagnosis of diabetes

No uncontrolled hypertension (diastolic 90 mmHg or below); based on British Hypertension Society guidance

No previous leg ulceration as a result of any cause

Non-smoker (but may have smoked in the past)

No intermittent claudication

No transient ischaemic attacks

No cerebral vascular accidents

No ischaemic heart disease

No diagnosis of rheumatoid arthritis

Ankle brachial pressure index: 0.9–1.2

These characteristics were then further refined by the steering group to form the inclusion criteria for the second stage of this study (*Table 4.1*).

Stage two

Ethical approval was obtained from East Suffolk local research ethics committee towards the end of 2003 based on the research question: 'Do patients wearing compression hosiery for leg problems other than past/present ulceration need a full assessment every 6 months?' However, early in 2004, the Research Consortium for East and West Suffolk NHS Trusts concluded that 'this extremely important piece of work' should be classed as clinical audit, not research. Initially, we felt frustrated having invested considerable time and effort since the issue was first raised, but we were determined to complete the project. Hence, the second stage of this study became a retrospective audit of nursing documentation for patients attending leg ulcer clinics within Suffolk Coastal PCT. A formal application to carry out a retrospective audit was submitted, approval was obtained and an audit tool was developed.

All data was collected historically from patients' initial assessment at leg ulcer clinics within the PCT and at subsequent reassessments until the audit date. Data spanned the period August 1998–1 August 2004 (6 years). Confidentiality was maintained by assigning a code to each patient. Using the inclusion criteria (see *Table 4.1*), the data collected for each patient wearing compression hosiery (class I or II) for reasons other than past or previous leg ulceration included:

- Date of birth (to determine age)
- Gender
- ABPI to right and left leg at each visit
- Blood pressure readings at each visit
- Any health status change and/or the development of diabetes at reassessment visits.

Results

A total of 101 patients met the inclusion criteria: 72 were female and 29 were male. Ages ranged from 39–92 years with a mean age of 71 years. From these

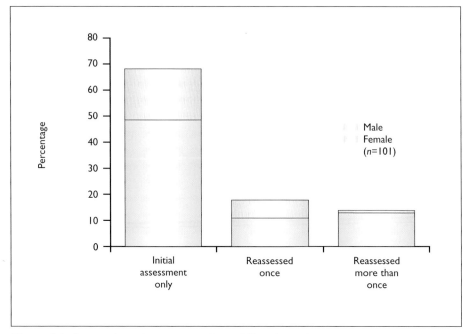

Figure 4.1: Comparisons between male and female patients

101 patients, 69 (68.3%) had an initial assessment, 18 (17.8%) had an initial assessment and one reassessment, and 14 (13.9%) had an initial assessment and two or more reassessments (*Figure 4.1*).

Of the patients assessed once only (*n*=69), the time period between the initial assessment and the data-collection point ranged from 1–72 months. As this was a retrospective audit with a flexible start date (based on the length of time a patient had been attending the leg clinic) but with a fixed end date, individuals with a short time scale had only recently started to attend the leg clinics. As there was no change to the health status for any patients in this study, it is likely that these patients had chosen not to attend for reassessment. However, a few patients may have stopped using compression hosiery or moved from the area and not informed the leg clinics; a minority may have died.

Of the patients reassessed once after their initial assessment (18 patients), five patients had that reassessment within 7 months. For the remaining patients in this group, the period between the initial assessment and reassessment ranged from 8–41 months. Fourteen patients were reassessed more than once: eight were reassessed twice; four were reassessed three times; and two were reassessed five times. Individuals who returned regularly for reassessment were probably responding to the advice given to all patients to attend for repeat Doppler assessments and new hosiery. As there was no health change for any of these patients, and Doppler readings varied only slightly, the extended periods between reassessment may reflect individual choice and professional feedback that all was well with their legs.

Data relating to ABPI readings showed only minimal variation. Thirty-two

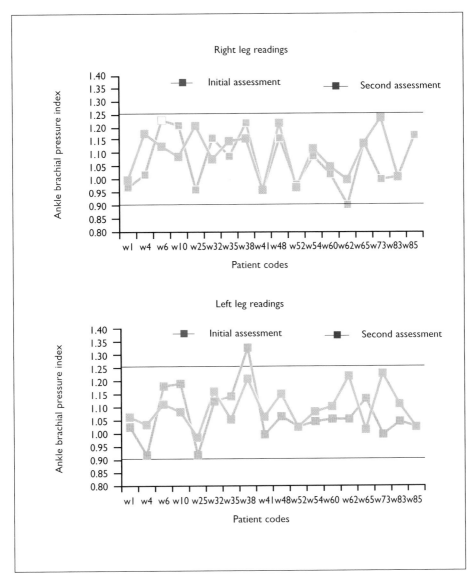

Figure 4.2: Doppler readings for patients who attended initial assessment and one reassessment

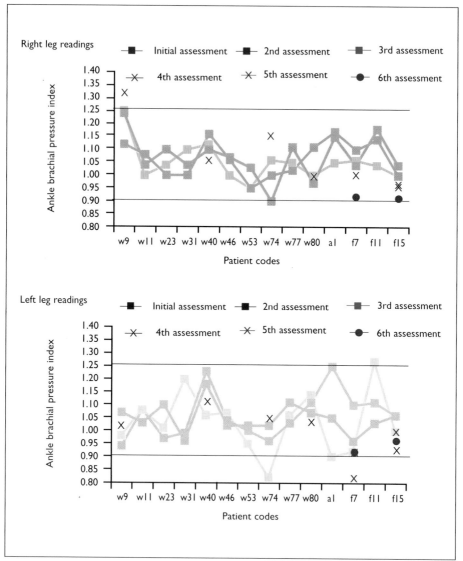

Figure 4.3: Doppler readings for patients who attended initial assessment and more than one reassessment

patients had Doppler readings at reassessment points, with only two patients showing a slight fall from the ABPI of 0.9 used as the inclusion criteria for this study (*Figures 4.2 and 4.3*).

Of the two patients showing a slight fall in ABPI, this only related to the reading for one leg and on one occasion for these patients. For both patients the subsequent readings returned to the inclusion criteria. Operator error may provide an explanation. At no point did the ABPI of any patient fall below 0.8. Taken together with no health status change, this demonstrates that all patients stayed within parameters generally considered safe for the use of prescribed compression hosiery. There were only minimal changes in diastolic blood pressure until patients were over 80 years of age, and then there was a gradual increase in diastolic blood pressure. However, for only one patient (reassessed once) did the diastolic blood pressure rise above 90 mmHg, the figure used as the inclusion criteria for this study.

Discussion

Although risk factors for arterial disease are well established (Vowden and Vowden, 1996; Herbert, 1997; Donnelly and London, 2000), indications of people whose ABPI may fall below the level considered safe to wear prescribed compression hosiery are unclear. The complete absence of research located on this topic led to the first stage of this study — a scrutiny of nursing documentation for 128 people wearing compression hosiery for leg problems other than past or present ulceration. Data was then analyzed and reviewed by a group of practitioners skilled in the care of leg ulcer patients. This strategy exposed for the first time the characteristics of people wearing compression hosiery for leg problems other than past or present ulceration. The ABPI for this group emerged as 0.9–1.2. These characteristics formed the inclusion criteria for the second stage of this study, a retrospective audit of nursing documentation for 101 patients who met these inclusion criteria from one PCT.

An ABPI of less than 0.8 is commonly regarded as a contraindication for high compression therapy (European Wound Management Association, 2003), with high compression bandage systems being the most common strategy to manage venous ulceration. An ABPI of 1.0–1.3 is considered indicative of normal arterial supply; 1.3 or above can represent a false high reading and is usually a result of the inability to compress adequately the arteries because of atherosclerosis (Ruff, 2003).

In the context of compression hosiery, external compression depends on the class of hosiery prescribed (class I, II or III). The severity of the underlying condition, dexterity and tolerance by the patient influences the classification of hosiery used, but the prevention of venous ulceration is best achieved by class III hosiery exerting in the region of 35-40 mmHg at the ankle (Edwards and Moffatt, 1996). Class I and II hosiery exert lower pressures, are indicated for mild oedema and varicose veins (Johnson, 2002) and represent the classification of compression hosiery used by all the patients in this study. At no time did the

ABPI of any patient in our study go outside the parameters of 0.8 and 1.3, when the wearing of compression hosiery would need to be reviewed but not necessarily discontinued (RCN, 1998; Vowden and Vowden, 2001).

Pankhurst (2004) attempted to address the question: 'At what point is wearing compression hosiery contraindicated by a reduction in ABPI?' Unfortunately, the author provides no information about the classification of compression hosiery worn by the patients. Based on 88 patients with healed venous leg ulcers, the conclusion reached is that repeat Doppler assessment for each patient with healed venous ulcers routinely at 3 months may be unnecessary and costly, and a staged approach to reassessment is suggested.

Poore et al (2002) report on a healed leg ulcer clinic using class II compression stockings where pedal pulses are checked at each patient visit (normally 6-monthly intervals); if faint or absent, or there are changes in the clinical picture, the ABPI is assessed. Only two patients with healed leg ulcers (from a study group of 96 patients) are indicated as having a reduction in ABPI over the period reviewed (2 years). However, palpating pedal pulses is not generally accepted practice, and inconsistencies between manual palpation and ABPI have been consistently demonstrated (Moffatt and O'Hare, 1995; RCN, 1998).

Another alternative, although currently not widely used, is the audible signal transmitted from a Doppler machine. A triphasic signal indicates normal arteries, a biphasic signal indicates some loss of elasticity as part of the ageing process, while a single sound or monophasic signal is indicative of vessel disease (Ruff, 2003).

Nationally, community nurses find it difficult to meet the recommended guidelines for reassessment of patients with leg ulceration, which includes Doppler ultrasound at 3-month intervals (Scottish Intercollegiate Guidelines Network, 1998) or 3- to 6-monthly based on local protocols (RCN, 1998), as a result of heavy clinical demands. This may be illustrated by the extended time periods between reassessments (2–32 months) for healed leg ulcers in Pankhurst's (2004) study. Patients appear to place much greater emphasis on attending for reassessment if they have, or have recently had, a leg ulcer. Extended time periods between reassessment (7-41 months) are evidenced in the audit reported in this article. However, in our study, patients were wearing hosiery for less clinical risk than to prevent venous ulcer reoccurrence as they had never had a venous ulcer. There is a considerably shorter period between reassessments for our patients with leg ulceration.

In our study, 68.3% of patients (69 patients) did not return for reassessment after initial assessment, measurement and prescription of compression hosiery for reasons other than leg ulceration. Pankhurst (2004) concludes that because healed leg ulcer patients were lost to follow-up (reassessment), this demonstrates how stable some patients' ABPI readings remain. In part this may be true. On the other hand, 14 patients (from a total of 110 patients with previous leg ulceration) no longer attended at the end of the first year in Poore et al's study (2002): five had died and nine were too frail to attend the hospital clinic. All our patients are carefully informed how to care for their legs and their hosiery at the initial assessment, and most patients probably felt sufficiently empowered to return to the clinic only if problems were experienced. No data are available to confirm this, but it needs to be borne in mind that none of our patients had ever had a leg ulcer, and many patients simply obtain replacement compression hosiery via a GP repeat prescription.

Of the 32 patients who did attend for reassessment, none had a change in their ABPI indicating compression hosiery should be discontinued, and only one had a diastolic blood pressure reading above 90 mmHg; both readings are indicative of arterial disease. However, for patients above the age of 80 years there was a small but gradual increase in diastolic blood pressure. This should be taken into consideration because age has a significant influence on the prevalence of peripheral arterial disease (Vowden and Vowden, 1996).

It is important to differentiate between patients with healed venous leg ulcers wearing prescribed compression hosiery to minimize the risk of ulcer reoccurrence, and patients wearing compression hosiery for 'well legs' (aching or swollen legs, or legs prone to varicose veins or deep vein thrombosis development). In Pankhurst's (2004) study, only 10 patients (study group 88 patients with healed venous ulceration) did not have past or current indications of arterial disease.

The carefully developed inclusion criteria for our study (see *Table 4.1*) meant that all 101 patients had no indication of arterial disease and had never had a leg ulcer. Significantly, there was no health status change, including the development of diabetes, for any patient during the 6-year period reviewed.

Conclusion

There have been significant changes to health care over recent years, influenced in part by scientific and medical developments, government policies and evidence-based practice (Department of Health, 1998; Gagan and Hewitt-Taylor, 2004). These drivers translate into increasing and competing demands on nursing time. Community practitioners now undertake many aspects of care that were previously the remit of doctors or nurses in acute care settings. At the same time, initiatives such as the 'expert patient' (Department of Health, 2001) have underlined patient empowerment, although this must be within an ethos of patient-centred care (RCN, 2004). Engaging with people to take greater responsibility for their health, increasing demands on community nurses' time and recognition that practice should be underpinned by credible evidence provides the backdrop to this report and subsequent recommendations.

The results of this study enable practitioners to review the care currently provided to people wearing prescribed compression hosiery for reasons other than to heal or prevent reoccurrence of venous leg ulceration. Following an initial detailed holistic assessment, including ABPI (a valuable screening tool for arterial disease (Vowden and Vowden, 2001)), those patients who meet identified characteristics (see *Table 4.1*) can, at the discretion of the professional prescribing the compression hosiery, be empowered to return for reassessment only if there is a change in their health status or skin changes to their legs. Replacement compression hosiery, normally every 6 months when wear is alternated between two pairs, would be via a repeat GP prescription. Critical to this recommendation is the health advice given to patients at initial assessment and the development of an information leaflet. Implementing these recommendations should enable community practitioners to meet some of the competing demands on their time without compromising the quality of care received by patients.

The authors would like to acknowledge the contributions of Val Moffatt, District Nurse, Suffolk Coastal Primary Care Trust, Tom Foster, Senior Lecturer, Suffolk College, Ipswich and Alan Norman, Clinical Audit Facilitator, East Suffolk Primary Care Trusts.

References

Department of Health (1998) *A First Class Service.* Department of Health, London

Department of Health (2001) *The Expert Patient: A New Approach to Chronic Disease Management for the 21st Century.* Department of Health, London

Donnelly R, London N, eds (2000) *ABC of Arterial and Venous Disease.* BMJ Books, London

Dowsett C (2004) Our agenda is to raise the standard of venous leg ulcer care. *J Wound Care* **13**(5): 181–5

Edwards L, Moffatt C (1996) The use of compression hosiery in the care of leg ulcers. *Nurs Stand* **10**(31): 53–6

European Wound Management Association (2003) *Understanding Compression Therapy.* Medical Education Partnership, London

Gagan M, Hewitt-Taylor J (2004) The issues for nurses involved in implementing evidence in practice. *Br J Nurs* **13**(20): 1216–20

Herbert L (1997) *Caring for the Vascular Patient.* Churchill Livingstone, New York

Johnson S (2002) Compression hosiery in the prevention and treatment of venous leg ulcers. *J Tissue Viabil* **12**(2): 67–74

Moffatt C, O'Hare L (1995) Ankle pulses are not sufficient to detect impaired arterial circulation in patients with leg ulcers. *J Wound Care* **4**(3): 134–8

Morrell C, Walters S, Dixon S, Collins K, Brereton L, Peters J, Brooker C (1998) Cost-effectiveness of community leg ulcer clinics: randomized controlled trial. *Br Med J* **316:** 1487–91

Nursing and Midwifery Council (2002a) *Code of Professional Conduct.* Nursing and Midwifery Council, London

Nursing and Midwifery Council (2002b) *Guidelines for Records and Record Keeping.* Nursing and Midwifery Council, London

Pankhurst S (2004) Should ABPI be reassured in patients with healed venous leg ulcers every three months? *J Wound Care* **13**(10): 438–40

Poore S, Cameron J, Cherry G (2002) Venous leg ulcer recurrence: prevention and healing. *J Wound Care* **11**(5): 197–9

Royal College of Nursing (1998) *The Management of Patients with Venous Leg Ulcers.* Clinical Practice Guidelines. Royal College of Nursing, London

Royal College of Nursing (2004) *The Future Nurse: The RCN Vision.* Royal College of Nursing, London (available from www.rcn.org.uk)

Ruff D (2003) Doppler assessment: calculating an ankle brachial pressure index. *Nurs Times* **99**(42): 62–5

Scottish Intercollegiate Guidelines Network (1998) *The Care of Patients with Chronic Leg Ulcers: A National Clinical Guideline.* SIGN, Edinburgh

Simon D, Freak L, Williams I, McCollum C (1994) Progression of arterial disease in patients with healed venous ulcers. *J Wound Care* **3**(4): 179–80

Vowden K, Vowden P (1996) Arterial disease: reversible and irreversible risk factors. *J Wound Care* **5**(2): 89–90

Vowden K, Vowden P (2001) Doppler and the ABPI: how good is our understanding? *J Wound Care* **10**(6): 197–201

Chapter 5

Uncommon causes of leg ulceration and lesions not to be missed

David Tillman

While most cases of leg ulceration are the result of venous and/or arterial disease and occur in older people, there are several other less common conditions that can lead to leg ulceration, often in younger people. This chapter examines the diagnosis and management of some of these conditions, almost all of which will require referral for specialist assessment and treatment.

Chronic leg ulcers constitute a major UK health problem, have a population prevalence of 1–3 per thousand, and occur mainly but not exclusively in older people. The aetiology in most patients is venous insufficiency (60–80%), with arterial disease being the major player in 10–30% of cases. A mixed aetiology is present in 10–20% of cases (Scottish Intercollegiate Guidelines Network (SIGN), 1998). The vast majority of patients are managed in the primary care setting, and in most cases diagnosis is not a problem.

There are a number of other, less common, causes of leg ulceration, which healthcare professionals should be aware of. In some of these conditions it is not uncommon for diagnosis and correct management to be delayed, resulting in increased morbidity. In addition, there are skin lesions that occur frequently on the leg that may cause significant problems for the patient if left untreated.

This chapter focuses on the diagnosis and appropriate management of some of these conditions.

Pyoderma gangrenosum

Pyoderma gangrenosum (PG) is a reactive, inflammatory, ulcerating skin condition of unknown aetiology. It is associated with an underlying systemic disease in up to 50% of cases. Rheumatoid arthritis, ulcerative colitis, Crohn's disease and haematological malignancy are among the most common disease associations (Wolff and Stingl, 2003).

PG typically begins as a painful, deep nodule or superficial pustule, which breaks down to form a painful ulcer. Onset may be accompanied by significant systemic disturbance and fever. Lesions occur at sites of minimal trauma in up to 20% of cases (Wolff and Stingl, 2003).

Diagnosis is based on the clinical appearance (*Figure 5.1*), which has three distinctive features:

■ A raised, purple edge
■ A necrotic, cribriform (sieve-like) base
■ An inflammatory flare.

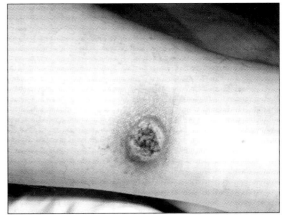

As the ulcer expands, the edge becomes undermined. Initially single, several other lesions often appear, with the legs, thighs and buttocks being the most commonly affected sites.

Figure 5.1: Pyoderma gangrenosum

Differential diagnosis includes other causes of ulceration such as infection, vasculitis, malignancy, insect bites and factitious ulceration. The main diagnostic error is to consider the initial lesion infective and thus to refer the patient only when the ulcer progresses despite antibiotic therapy, or when additional lesions appear. If there is diagnostic doubt, a biopsy should be performed, but histology of PG is not specific.

The course of the disease is variable, and when present often follows that of the underlying condition. Healing often results in atrophic scarring, which may be disfiguring.

Treatment should be aimed at the skin manifestations of PG and any underlying disease. For mild skin lesions, topical or intralesional steroid injections may be used. Newer topical agents, such as tacrolimus, have also produced good results in early lesions (Reich et al, 1998; Petering et al, 2001). Surgical debridement or excision should be avoided as this may trigger new lesions.

In moderate or severe disease, systemic therapy is required. Oral prednisolone is usually effective, but initial high doses of 40–100 mg daily may be required, necessitating the use of steroid-sparing immunosuppressive agents.

Necrobiosis lipoidica

Necrobiosis lipoidica (NL) is a condition that occurs chiefly, but not exclusively, in patients with diabetes mellitus, and is three times more common in women. The classic clinical picture of NL is the appearance of one or more sharply demarcated yellow-brown plaques on the shins (*Figure 5.2*). It may start on one leg but is eventually almost always bilateral. The skin becomes atrophic, smooth and shiny, with loss of skin appendages, including hair follicles. In fully developed lesions, dermal blood vessels are easily seen (telangiectasia), and in 13–35% of cases ulceration occurs. The mean age of onset is around 30 years old. In patients with diabetes, the degree of hyperglycaemia and diabetic control do not correlate with the presence of NL (Bub and Olerud, 2003).

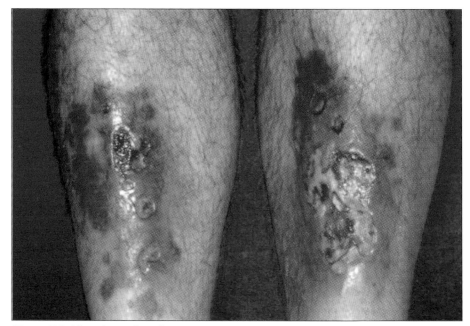

Figure 5.2: Necrobiosis lipoidica

The disease often runs a protracted course but does tend to burn itself out with time. Topical steroids used early might slow progression. The focus should be on the prevention of ulcers. When ulceration does occur, the same wound care principles apply as for diabetic ulcers.

Vasculitis

Cutaneous vasculitis is a well recognized, albeit uncommon, cause of leg ulceration. It presents with multiple, palpable, purpuric (non-blanching on pressure) lesions on the legs, which are often more numerous distally (*Figure 5.3*).

Lesions often coalesce to form larger areas of damaged skin, skin

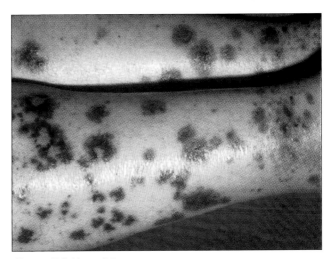

Figure 5.3: Vasculitic puroura

necrosis and ulceration. There are many underlying causes of vasculitis, but the most common are connective tissue diseases such as rheumatoid arthritis and systemic lupus erythematosus, medication, underlying infection (especially streptococcal) and several haematological conditions.

In many instances, vasculitis is confined to the skin, but screening for systemic involvement – particularly renal disease – is required. Treatment is aimed at the underlying medical condition.

Erythema induratum

Erythema induratum is an uncommon, but well recognized, cause of leg ulceration. It mainly affects young or middle-aged women with poor circulation. In many cases there is an association with tuberculosis.

Clinically, multiple ulcers appear, mainly on the back of the legs, often with surrounding inflammation (*Figure 5.4*). The disease is caused by inflammation in subcutaneous fat (panniculitis). Management of these patients requires investigation for other causes of panniculitis and screening for tuberculosis. The disease responds to antituberculosis therapy.

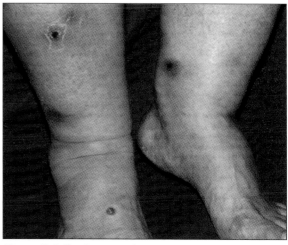

Figure 5.4: Erythema induratum

Cellulitis

Cellulitis is a fairly common condition that erupts acutely and can be recurrent. It is most commonly unilateral, a major differentiating feature from contact dermatitis to dressings, which is usually bilateral. Patients often experience premonitory symptoms of malaise and influenza-like symptoms in the 24 hours before the leg becomes red, hot, swollen and painful (*Figure 5.5*).

Risk factors include obesity, diabetes, venous stasis, tinea pedis and a previous episode of cellulitis. There can be lymphangitis and tender inguinal lymphadenopathy.

If the skin texture is normal, the infective organism is highly likely to be *Streptococcus spp.*

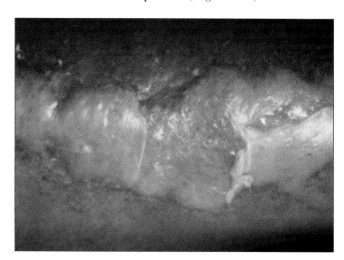

Figure 5.5: Cellulitis

If, however, there is epidermal damage with serous exudation and honey-coloured crusting, *Staphylococcus aureus* is present and has to be treated. The extent of redness in the leg itself may increase after antibiotic treatment is commenced. Patient assessment should, however, be mainly based on symptoms, temperature and colour and temperature of the first affected area of involvement. If all these are improving, a change in antibiotic therapy is rarely indicated.

Treatment of mild cellulitis in an otherwise well patient is phenoxymethyl penicillin (penicillin V), 500 mg four times daily. Treatment duration depends on response, but up to 4 weeks may be required. Erythromycin and clindamycin are effective in penicillin–allergic individuals. If the infection is moderate to severe, admission and treatment with intravenous benzylpenicillin, 1.2 g four times a day, is the treatment of choice (Weinberg et al, 2003). If, in addition, the skin is broken and ulcerated and there is concern about *S. aureus*, flucloxacillin will be added.

Bullous pemphigoid

Bullous pemphigoid is a blistering condition, which is more common in patients over 60 years of age. The most common site of onset is the lower limb.

It is usually bilateral and fairly symmetrical. On a background of normal or areas of inflamed skin, large tense blisters, some of which may be haemorrhagic, appear acutely (*Figure 5.6*).

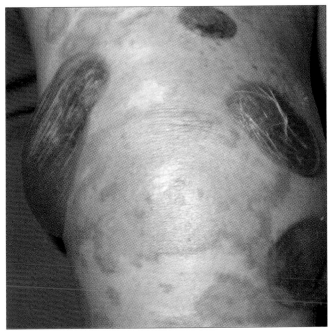

Figure 5.6: Bullous pemphigoid

The major differential diagnoses include insect bites and a drug eruption. Diagnosis is clinched with a skin biopsy, which is sent for routine pathology (haematoxylin and eosin staining), together with direct immunofluorescence. The blister is the result of a split in the skin at the junction between the epidermis and dermis. The condition is usually idiopathic, with no identifiable reason for the immunological attack on the skin (Wojnarowska et al, 2004).

Treatment is with topical steroids if the disease is mild, but in most instances systemic prednisolone is required at initial doses of 60–100 mg, with the addition of steroid-sparing agents as the steroid dose is tapered (Burns et al, 2004).

Skin cancer

Although skin cancer does not often cause leg ulceration, it can do so and should not be ignored as a possible cause. In addition, nursing practitioners should become familiar with potentially dangerous lesions that can occur on the leg as well as on other body sites. These include Bowen's disease, squamous cell carcinoma and melanoma.

Bowen's disease

This condition represents squamous cell carcinoma *in situ* and is not uncommon in older people, particularly in women. It usually presents as a superficial scaly plaque, which may be irregular in shape. The most common site is the leg (*Figure 5.7*). In many cases, multiple lesions are present. Fortunately, the disease tends to spread laterally within the epidermis, and only in more longstanding or neglected cases does invasive squamous carcinoma develop. If there is doubt about

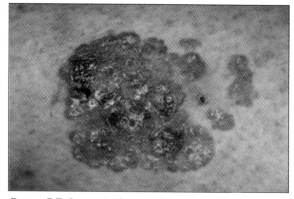

Figure 5.7: Bowen's disease

diagnosis or if dermal invasion is suspected, a diagnostic biopsy is required. Treatment options include excision (especially for small lesions), cryotherapy with liquid nitrogen and the newer modality, photodynamic therapy.

Squamous cell carcinoma

Squamous cell carcinoma (SCC) (*Figure 5.8*) is the second most common skin cancer after basal cell carcinoma (Grossman and Leffell, 2003), the latter not commonly seen on the leg.

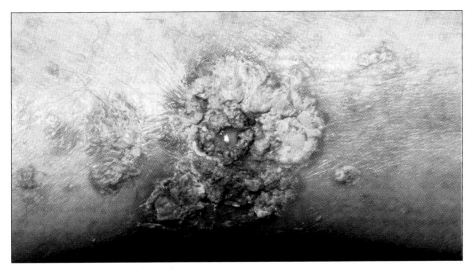

Figure 5.8: Squamous cell carcinoma

It presents as a growing keratotic lesion that may ulcerate and become secondarily infected. The major risk factor for the development of SCC is the cumulative amount of ultraviolet light exposure, and for this reason it often arises on a background of obvious sun damage. Additionally, SCC of the leg is more common in women. SCC is also more common in older patients (a sharp increase in incidence is seen after the age of 40 years), and fair-skinned individuals are at highest risk (Grossman and Leffell, 2003). Patients with psoriasis who have had high doses of photochemotherapy have a 30-fold increased risk of non-melanoma skin cancer, most of which are SCCs (Stern and Lange, 1988); in transplant patients, who are immunosuppressed, the risk is increased 18 times (Gupta et al, 1986). Such patients require close follow-up as they may develop multiple lesions.

Invasive squamous carcinoma can arise from an actinic keratosis or an area of Bowen's disease. It can also occur in a chronic leg ulcer. For this reason, a biopsy of a chronic leg ulcer should be arranged if the appearance of the edge becomes raised.

Treatment is by excision and in early lesions is curative. If neglected, SCC can spread, usually initially to draining lymph nodes, in this case in the groin. Radiotherapy is an alternative treatment.

Melanoma

Over a 20-year period between 1979–98 the incidence of melanoma per 100 000 population per year in Scotland increased from 3.5 to 10.6 in men, and from 7.0 to 13.1 in women (MacKie et al, 2002). Fortunately this trend is not continuing in women, where incidence is beginning to plateau, but the rise in incidence in men continues (MacKie et al, 2002). As this skin cancer is potentially fatal, all medical professionals should be able to recognize suspicious signs in a pigmented skin lesion requiring referral for an expert opinion.

The major signs of early melanoma are a change in size, shape or colour of a naevus (mole) or pigmented skin lesion. Even if there is no history of change, irregularity in colour and/or shape of a lesion is a worrying feature, particularly if the border is like the contours of a map (*Figure 5.9a*) or the lesion is two-tone ('half-and-half') in colour (*Figure 5.9b*).

Figure 5.9: Melanoma: a) map-like contoured edge; b) bi-coloured lesion

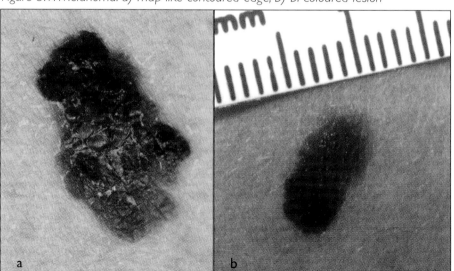

Symptoms such as itching, crusting or bleeding are also an indication to rigorously assess the lesion. The major determinant of prognosis is the tumour thickness, determined by biopsy. If the lesion has ulcerated, the prognosis is less favourable.

Treatment involves excision with an appropriate margin of normal skin, and sentinel node biopsy is now carried out if the primary lesion is over 1 mm in thickness.

Conclusion

Although most leg ulcers are caused by circulatory problems, community nurses will occasionally be presented with an ulcer with a different aetiology. Nurses should take the time to familiarize themselves with the signs and symptoms of the different presentations, and to make the appropriate referrals for further investigation and treatment.

References

Bub JL, Olerud JE (2003) Diabetes mellitus. In: Freeberg IM, Eisen AZ, Wolf K, Austen KF, Goldsmith LA, Katz SI, eds. *Fitzpatrick's Dermatology in General Medicine*. 6th edn. McGraw-Hill, New York: 1651–61

Burns T, Breathnach S, Cox N, Griffiths C (2004) *Rook's Textbook of Dermatology*. 7th edn. Blackwell Publishing, Oxford

Grossman D, Leffell DJ (2003) Squamous cell carcinoma. In: Freeberg IM, Eisen AZ, Wolf K, Austen KF, Goldsmith LA, Katz SI, eds. *Fitzpatrick's Dermatology in General Medicine*. 6th edn. McGraw-Hill, New York: 737–47

Gupta AK, Cardella CJ, Haberman HF (1986) Cutaneous malignant neoplasms in patients with renal transplants. *Arch Dermatol* **122**(11): 1288–93

MacKie RM, Bray CA, Hole DJ et al (2002) Incidence of and survival from malignant melanoma in Scotland: an epidemiological study. *Lancet* **360**(9333): 587–91

Petering H, Kiehl P, Breuer C et al (2001) Pyoderma gangrenosum: successful topical therapy with tacrolimus (FK506). *Hautarzt* **52:** 47–50

Reich K, Vente C, Neumann C (1998) Topical tacrolimus for pyoderma gangrenosum. *Br J Dermatol* **139**(4): 755–7

Scottish Intercollegiate Guidelines Network (1998) *The Care of Patients with Chronic Leg Ulcer. A National Clinical Guideline.* SIGN, Edinburgh

Stern RS, Lange R (1988) Non-melanoma skin cancer occurring in patients treated with PUVA five to ten years after first treatment. *J Invest Dermatol* **92**(2): 120–4

Weinberg MN, Swartz AN, Tsao H, Johnson RA (2003) Soft tissue infections: erysipelas, cellulitis, gangrenous cellulitis and myonecrosis. In: Freeberg IM, Eisen AZ, Wolf K, Austen KF, Goldsmith LA, Katz SI, eds. *Fitzpatrick's Dermatology in General Medicine.* 6th edn. McGraw-Hill, New York: 1883–95

Wojnarowska F, Venning VA, Burge SM (2004) Immunobullous diseases. In: Burns T, Breathnach S, Cox N, Griffiths C, eds. *Rook's Textbook of Dermatology.* 7th edn. Blackwell Publishing, Oxford: 41.25–41.35

Wolff K, Stingl G (2003) Pyoderma gangrenosum. In: Freeberg IM, Eisen AZ, Wolf K, Austen KF, Goldsmith LA, Katz SI, eds. *Fitzpatrick's Dermatology in General Medicine.* 6th edn. McGraw-Hill, New York: 969–76

Chapter 6

The Lindsay Leg Club® Model: a model for evidence-based leg ulcer management

Ellie Lindsay

Leg Club® is a unique model of community-based leg ulcer care. By providing nursing care in a non-medical, social environment, the model has several benefits: it removes the stigma associated with leg ulcers and helps isolated older people reintegrate into their communities, which in turn improves concordance and has a positive impact on healing and recurrence rates. In an atmosphere of de-stigmatization, empathy and peer support, positive health beliefs are promoted and patients take ownership of their treatment. The Leg Club model creates a framework in which nurses, patients and local community can collaborate as partners in the provision of holistic care. The model also provides an environment for appropriate supportive education, advice and information.

For many older people living in the community, loneliness is a significant issue. Retirement, poor mobility, the death of family or friends, or the effects of demographic change on the cohesiveness of the family unit can all create an environment of social isolation. For older people suffering from leg ulcers, this isolation is often heightened, and can have detrimental effects on their health. Pain, odour and obtrusive bandages may exacerbate feelings of low self-esteem, depression and social stigma, which in turn can lead to poor concordance with treatment and low healing rates (Lindsay, 2000). Even when healing is achieved, poor concordance leads to high levels of recurrence.

Health beliefs play an important role when treating and managing patients with leg ulcers. One of the main problems the district nurse is confronted with when treating a patient in his/her own home, is poor concordance with treatment. As Becker (1974) asserted, even when an individual recognizes personal susceptibility (e.g. to leg ulceration), action will not occur unless he/she also believes that becoming ill will bring organic or social repercussions. So in an already isolated individual, the social repercussions are negligible, and motivation to act can therefore be low.

It has also been claimed that a lack of an informal support network may result in patients becoming psychologically dependant on healthcare professionals (Poulton, 1991). Poulton further highlighted the importance of an holistic assessment, taking into account both the psychological and social factors of the patient's situation and being proactive in organizing other social contacts for the patient.

As a district nurse in Suffolk, I was aware of anecdotal evidence that social factors and isolation could significantly influence patients' response to treatment. Further enquiry (via literature review, examination of demographic factors and patients' daily circumstances, and a study of established leg ulcer clinics) led to the conclusion that a new type of clinic could help to address these issues. The conceptual framework for this new approach was a health belief model (Becker and Maiman, 1975), for obtaining and assessing the patient's views and perception of health and well-being. The model addresses the individual's concerns, motivating factors, demographic issues, attitudes, interactions and enabling factors. Becker (1974) introduced self-efficacy into the health belief model, and identified an association between belief in the treatment, motivation and concordance. The model assumes that wellbeing is a common objective for all, and that locus of control is associated with mastery of health information, motivation, effective problem solving, sense of responsibility and desire for active participation in health care.

The achievement of the desired degree of excellence in nursing practice demands an appraisal of the new pattern of nursing service organized around the concept of progressive patient empowerment. The ultimate goal of the community nurse practitioner is to function professionally, educatively, therapeutically and creatively. To achieve this paradigm, the clinician must be given the freedom and assistance needed to develop his/her unique role in the patient's therapeutic care. Nursing services can either facilitate or block educative-therapeutic nursing, depending on the goals and philosophy of the nursing service leadership.

In the author's experience, obstruction and opposition were to be a constant factor in introducing this new concept of leg ulcer management within her practice community. It was evident that nurses (and higher tiers of management) are strongly polarized in reaction to the prospect of change. There are many who are open to examine the evidence, who are challenged and who are motivated by the potential for improving care delivery through innovation. They may already be leaders within their working community or recently qualified nurses with fresh idealism and the motivation to influence those around them. Conversely, there are those who interpret any proposal for change as a criticism of their longstanding practice, particularly when that change involves a perceived loss of 'status' associated with patient empowerment. Despite resistance and lack of support from some quarters, the first clinic to be based on the principles set out by the author were established in a rural community in 1995.

How a Leg Club® works

Leg Clubs® were conceived as a unique partnership between community nurses, patients and the local community to provide leg ulcer management in a social, non-medical setting. In accordance with the themes of the *NHS Plan* (Department of Health, 2001) and clinical governance, patients are empowered with a sense of ownership and recognition that they are stakeholders in their own treatment. Emphasis is placed on social interaction, participation, empathy and peer support.

A Leg Club is characterized by four features that differentiate it from conventional leg ulcer clinics:

- It is community-based and held in a non-medical setting, such as a village/community centre, church hall or meeting room (e.g. *Figure 6.1*)
- Patients are treated collectively (*Figure 6.2*)
- It operates on a drop-in basis (no appointments required)
- It incorporates a fully-integrated, 'well leg' regimen. The practice of

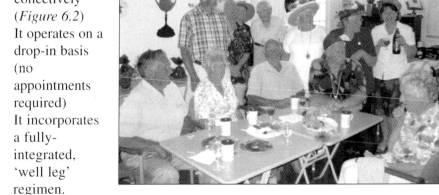

Figure 6.1: Leg Club® meeting

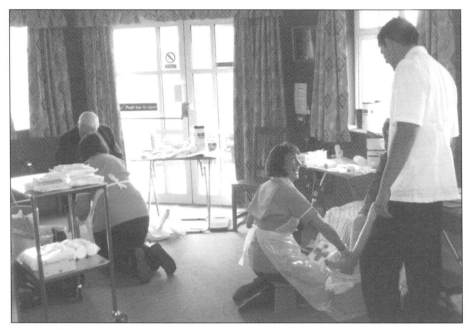

Figure 6.2: Patients are treated collectively

treating patients in isolation restricts the opportunity for peer support and education, and reinforces feelings of stigma that an individual may already be experiencing. In Leg Clubs, care is delivered collectively in a social, non-medical environment that facilitates socialization and peer support and empowers patients to participate in, and take ownership of, their treatment. In such an environment, example setting and role model emulation can flourish, providing powerful influences to help modify beliefs and change behaviour in non-concordant patients — influences that are not present in the typical one-to-one 'nurse dominant/patient passive' relationship.

However, collective working can be extremely challenging for some nurses, although objections are typically a nursing perception, not an issue for patients. The receptionist and staff explain the collective treatment regimen to new patients and ensure that provision is available for individual treatment should it be requested. To date, no patient has objected to being treated collectively and no incidents of cross-infection have occurred within the author's experience.

The principal aims of the Leg Club are therefore to:

- Empower patients to become stakeholders in their own treatment, promoting a sense of ownership and involvement
- Meet the social needs of isolated patients by providing a mechanism for social interaction, empathy and peer support

- Rebuild patients' self-esteem and self-respect by de-stigmatizing their condition
- Facilitate an informal support network
- Achieve concordance to treatment through informed beliefs and modified behaviour
- Provide continuity of care and a coordinated team approach to its delivery
- Minimize recurrence by systematic post-treatment monitoring and 'well leg' checks
- Adopt a simple, flexible drop-in approach that encourages attendance for information and advice, facilitating early diagnosis of problems
- Provide an informal forum for opportunistic health promotion and education.

Leg Clubs are not 'owned' by a healthcare provider, but by the local community. They provide a community-based venue at which patients (referred to in the Clubs as 'members') may elect to meet and attend for treatment. They are not intended to replace existing care delivery mechanisms but to complement them by responding to both the clinical and psychosocial needs of members. Apart from the direct costs of care delivery, Leg Clubs are self-funded (running costs and equipment costs) through money raised by volunteers within the community. In setting up Leg Clubs, nurses truly 'get to know' the communities they serve, working alongside the community and members to provide an environment of genuine patient empowerment.

The Leg Club model incorporates strict criteria governing environment and clinical practice, defined in written guidelines and comprehensive documentation. Defined safe working practices, covering areas such as infection control, risk analysis and the use of equipment, must be implemented before the opening of any new venue. Clinics are subsequently subject to regular audit to ensure continued adherence to Leg Club standards and enable comparative benchmarking to be undertaken. Routine data collection and analysis is a vital component of the model as it provides a measurement tool for clinicians to identify opportunities for continual improvement and sustained best practice.

Only clinics adhering to the Leg Club model and practicing to its prescribed standards are entitled to use the Leg Club title. To prevent the title being employed inappropriately, it is protected by a Registered Trade Mark (®).

The impact of Leg Clubs

Statistical data have been collected and independently analyzed since the inception of the first Leg Club. An ethnographic study identified patients' positive attitudes and a strong sense of ownership in 'their' club (Lindsay, 1996). Clinically, non-concordance to treatment was virtually eliminated and there was evidence of higher healing rates, illustrated by many members whose long-standing ulcers either healed or greatly improved as a direct result of this change in approach.

It was evident that before attending the clinic some of the members had been aware of the severity of their ulcers and the need for treatment, but had not been concordant with it because they felt some antipathy towards the medical establishment.

Some members disclosed that their attitude to their problems and treatment had undergone change as a result of knowledge they had acquired in the Club environment. Through awareness of their own and others' problems, they had become involved in related issues pertaining to their treatment and expected outcome. Their greater knowledge had led to an improved sense of self-worth and a belief that they were enabled to participate in their own treatment and care. The social aspects associated with their care emerged as the key factor in the healing process, and the clinical treatment became secondary. It was stimulating to observe how well individuals respond to an holistic approach to their care, and the empowerment associated with that approach.

Prophylaxis

The 'well leg' programme of the Leg Club model is aimed at prophylaxis education and advice, and prevention and maintenance of further leg-related problems once an ulcer has healed. According to McAllister and Farquhar (1992), health beliefs have important implications for nursing given the role of the nurse in health promotion and patient teaching. Although primarily targeted at the older population, the informal nature of the clinic has encouraged patients as young as 19 years to attend for advice and treatment, creating opportunities for early diagnosis, education and health promotion (Lindsay, 2000).

People's willingness to attend for 'well leg' checks and ongoing health education has resulted in a dramatic reduction in the incidence and recurrence of leg ulcers to <4% per annum. This compares favourably with data from various studies demonstrating high recurrence rates for leg ulceration. For example, Callam et al (1985) undertook a survey of 600 patients with 827 ulcerated legs of which 67% had recurrent ulcers, 35% of whom had experienced four or more episodes of ulceration. The low recurrence rates associated with Leg Clubs support the rationale of patient empowerment and the synergistic effect of ongoing health promotion and education in an integrated well-leg regimen.

Members' feedback

A small survey was designed by the chairman and committee of Grundisburgh Leg Club to obtain their members' views of the two local Leg Clubs. The survey was conducted by both Grundisburgh and Debenham Leg Club committee members, and the findings were collated and analyzed by a statistician.

The survey indicated that a non-threatening environment was an important factor of the Clubs' success. The members commented on their reluctance to visit a medical centre for treatment, but found that attending a clinic in a social setting gave them a sense of purpose, a feeling that they shared a common problem and that they were not in isolation. The data further identified that they formed friendships and gained an understanding of others' problems and needs, and their medically-related problems became secondary. Through this network of mutual support and friendship, concordance to treatment resulted from a strong sense of motivation. This was expressed through their trust in one another, confidence in themselves and understanding of their own treatment.

Local involvement

Another interesting facet of the Leg Club model has been the development of roles within the local community volunteer group. In many parts of the world, retired people are seen as active individuals who participate in neighbourhood committees, educational activities, welfare work and serving their neighbourhood in various ways. Therefore it is interesting to note that the majority of the Leg Club teams have community volunteers from this group who have elected to transfer from retirement status to become an extremely productive resource contributing to their community. Far from categorizing retired people as a frail, incapacitated or dependant group, the Leg Club model provides a framework in which older members of the community have an opportunity to play a valued and fulfilling role in their community and remain as active as possible. Their enthusiasm and energy has resulted in the creation of friendship clubs and peer groups where support and advice is offered to volunteers involved in newly formed Leg Clubs. The role of the volunteer receptionist has evolved to include newsletters, questionnaires, general information, fund-raising letters and information leaflets, organization of fund-raising events, maintenance of member registers and documentation. Two committee volunteers have successfully applied for substantial awards from the National Lottery. As one volunteer stated, 'I never thought life began at 84'!

Leg Club roll-out

Leg Clubs have been facilitated and opened around the UK — in Dorset, Suffolk, Norfolk, Gloustershire, Worstershire, West and East Sussex and Essex. Many more are currently at the embryonic stage in England, Scotland and Wales, planning to open during 2005. There are currently four Leg Clubs in Australia — in Adelaide, Brisbane and the Gold Coast. The concept has been disseminated in the UK and overseas through journals, conference presentations and seminars, and is a past winner of a *British Journal of Nursing (BJN)* Clinical Practice Award and *Nursing Standard* Nurse 2003 Award (Wound Care).

Nursing teams that have taken on this method of care delivery, working in an open culture, have reported not only improved patient outcomes, but also greatly enhanced teamworking and morale. In addition, a number of early adopters have received awards for their work including, in the current year, *BJN* Awards for Wound Care (runner-up) and Compression Therapy (winner), and two NHS Trust Innovation awards.

Furthermore, a recent study (Edwards et al, 2005a) has clearly shown that the provision of a Leg Club model of care promotes improved ulcer healing and decreased levels of pain in clients with chronic venous leg ulcers.

Successful Leg Clubs are the product of competent, open minded and motivated nursing teams working to best-practice guidelines with local health organization management support. However, patient empowerment is not an easy concept, and it is inevitable that some nurses and nurse managers are uncomfortable with the notion of moving from a 'nurse dominant/patient passive' relationship to one of an equal partnership in care.

Ultimately, change must be supported and enshrined in management policy if it is to prove sustainable in the face of loss of key motivated personnel. In the absence of senior management support and encouragement, Leg Clubs are dependant on the commitment and motivation of individual nurses; therefore even the most successful are vulnerable to staff changes. New staff, lacking management direction, understanding and ownership are unlikely to provide essential continuity. It is interesting to note that, in the majority of cases, those most vocal in opposition have never visited a Leg Club to observe the excellent work being done for patients who are de-stigmatized and collectively treated in an open, social environment. Patient quality of life is not a consideration that is cited in their arguments.

Current developments

In 2002, Queensland University of Technology was awarded a nursing research grant to undertake a 2-year, randomized, control study with St Luke's Community Nursing Service, replicating the Leg Club model. The study aimed to examine the effectiveness of a community Leg Club intervention in improving healing rates, quality of life, health status, levels of pain, functional ability and the model's cost-effectiveness of care. Courtney et al (2004) demonstrated that the data collected indicated that significant improvements in all areas had been achieved in the intervention group. In their pilot study report, Edwards et al (2005b) concluded that a community Leg Club environment provided added benefits apart from wound care expertise and evidence-based care; knowledge gained from the study provided evidence to guide service delivery and improve patient outcomes.

Documentation is the cornerstone to delivering evidence-based care. A software programme is currently under development to facilitate completion and analysis of the comprehensive Leg Club practice documentation. To ensure that prescribed procedures and standards are achieved and maintained throughout the Leg Club network, a comprehensive, 32-page audit tool has been compiled and employed.

Researchers from the Royal College of Nursing are undertaking a national audit of venous leg ulcers, funded by the Commission for Health Improvement. Leg Clubs are to be included in this project, and selected Leg Clubs will participate in the audit programme. Researchers also plan to meet Leg Club members to discuss the role of expert patient groups (Department of Health, 2001).

Conclusion

Leg Clubs have been shown to provide tangible benefits for all involved in the delivery of leg ulcer management:

- Significant cost savings for the healthcare provider
- An environment of truly holistic care for patients
- An enhanced and productive nursing/community relationship
- A forum for health promotion and education
- An accessible setting for opportunistic early detection and treatment.

References

Becker M (1974) The health belief model and sick role behaviour. *Proceedings of a Workshop/Symposium on Compliance with Therapeutic Regimens.* McMaster University, Hamilton, Ontario, Canada

Becker M, Maiman L (1975) Sociobehavioural determinants of compliance with health and medical care recommendations. *Medical Care* **13**(1): 10–25

Callam H, Ruckley C, Harper D, Dale J (1985) Chronic ulceration of the leg: extent of the problem and provision of care. *Br Med J* **290**: 1855–6

Courtney M, Edwards H, Finlayson K, Lindsay E, Lewis C, Dumble J (2004) *Randomised Controlled Trail of a Community Nursing Intervention for Managing Chronic Venous Leg Ulcers.* Poster presented at AWMA, Tasmania and International Research Conference, Cambridge, UK

Edwards H, Courtney M, Finlayson K et al (2005a) Chronic venous leg ulcers: effect of a community nursing intervention on pain and healing. *Nurs Standard* **19**(52): 47–54

Edwards H, Courtney M, Finlayson K, Lewis C, Lindsay E, Dumble J (2005b) Improved healing rates for chronic venous leg ulcers: pilot study results from a randomized controlled trial of a community nursing intervention. *Int J Nurs Pract* **11**: 169–76

Department of Health (2001) *The Expert Patient – A New Approach to Chronic Disease Management.* Department of Health, London

Lindsay E (1996) *What are Patients' Views of Leg Ulcer Management in a Social Community Clinic?* BSc dissertation, University College Suffolk

Lindsay E (2000) Leg clubs: a new approach to patient-centred leg ulcer management. *Nurs Health Sci* **2**(3): 139–41

McAllister G, Farquhar M (1992) Health beliefs: a cultural division? *J Adv Nurs* **17**(12): 1447–54

Poulton B (1991) Factors influencing patient compliance. *Nurs Stand* **5**(36): 3–5

Chapter 7

Clinical variance in assessing risk of pressure ulcer development

C Sharp, G Burr, M Broadbent, M Cummins, H Casey, A Merriman

Nurses working in one area health service (AHS) in Sydney, Australia, expressed concern about the development of pressure ulcers in hospitalized patients. Anecdotal evidence suggested that a variety of approaches were being used to assess patients to identify those at risk of pressure ulcer development. A questionnaire was distributed to all registered nurses (*n*=2113) in clinical settings within the AHS. Data was analyzed using frequency distribution. The response rate was 40% (*n*=850), of which 444 were useable. Nurses generally do not use a tool to assess pressure ulcer risk potential, but rely on a range of practice procedures and risk indicators. It is recommended that a pressure ulcer project group be established to evaluate existing tools, or if necessary to develop a tool for the assessment of patients to identify those at risk of developing pressure ulcers.

In 1997, a group of nurses working in a major area health service (AHS) in Sydney, Australia, expressed concern about the development of pressure ulcers (PUs) in the patients being cared for in their hospitals. At that time there were no Australian guidelines for the prevention of PUs, and anecdotal evidence suggested that a variety of approaches were being used to assess patients to identify those at risk of PU development.

With the establishment of the Nursing Research Centre for Adaptation in Health and Illness (NRCAHI) at the University of Sydney, Australia, an opportunity arose for representatives from the health facilities in the AHS and NRCAHI to investigate collaboratively the apparent clinical variance. The first stage in the project was to establish current practice in PU assessment, prevention and care.

Literature review

There is a vast collection of literature on PUs, both in Australia and overseas; however, valid information on the assessment of patients to identify those at risk of developing PUs is sparse (Exton-Smith, 1987; Callaghan, 1994; Pearson, 1997). Although several risk-assessment tools are available, little research exists to support their reliability and validity (Fletcher, 1997; Hoskins and Ramstadius, 1998; Quickfall and Shields, 1998), and they are not widely used in the particular AHS in the investigation (Sharp et al, 2000). It is generally accepted, however, that PUs occur in patients with limited mobility (Exton-Smith and Sherwin, 1961; Hibbs, 1982; Allman et al, 1986; Versluysen, 1986; Exton-Smith, 1987; Crow, 1988; Hawthorn and Nyquist, 1988; Bliss, 1999; Schoonhoven et al, 2002), and in those who are unable to feel, or respond by moving, to local pain and pressure (Versluysen, 1986; Bliss, 1999; Schoonhoven et al, 2002).

Previous research has focused on the incidence and prevalence of PUs (Ramstadius, 1994; Klei et al, 1997; Pearson, 1997) and on specific intervention modalities (Curry and Casady, 1992; Lockyer-Stevens, 1993; Jiricka et al, 1995; Whittle et al, 1996; Boettger, 1997; Zernicke, 1997; Waterlow, 1998). In New South Wales in 1993, prevalence rates of 3% and 17% were reported (Ramstadius, 1994) and in South Australia, 4% (Pearson, 1997); while in Victoria a 1995 survey of 30 nursing homes and a major teaching hospital revealed prevalence rates of between 5% and 10% (Klei et al, 1997).

The annual cost in Australia for treating PUs is estimated to be as much as $350 million (Klei et al, 1997), with the cost of treating just one patient with a stage four PU, not including the cost of the admitting condition, estimated at $61 230 (Young, 1997).

Traditionally, the responsibility for PU prevention has been with nurses, who may be held accountable for the quality of care they deliver. As the Australian population becomes more litigious, nurses may be subject to legal action if a patient develops a PU during a hospital stay (Dimond, 1994). Therefore, assessment of patients is paramount so that interventions for prevention are put in place for those at risk.

AHS policy review

The researchers felt that it was necessary to identify the varied methods used by nurses in the AHS to establish baseline information from which further research could be undertaken. It was felt that if patients were assessed for risk, much of the physical and emotional cost to the patient as well as the nursing time and resources devoted to wound management for PUs could be avoided. A review of policy documentation revealed that there were gross inconsistencies between hospitals in the AHS. Some policy documents contained information about manual-handling risks, offering patients bedpans or urinals, repositioning patients and ensuring that patients are comfortable. However, they do not mention when or how assessment should occur or what to do if a patient is deemed to be at risk of PU development, or indeed if a PU develops. In contrast, the policy at another hospital in the AHS states that the Norton Scale (Norton, 1996) is to be used to assess all patients on admission. Patients deemed to be at risk are then referred to the appropriate clinical nurse consultant. The policies at yet another two hospitals in the same AHS do not include assessment of PU risk, nor is there a risk-assessment tool. However, both of these hospitals have instructions for the documentation of PUs once they occur.

The study

Study design

An exploratory descriptive research design using a survey questionnaire was conducted to answer the following research question: 'What is current nursing practice within the AHS to assess patients' risk of PU development?'

Method

A survey questionnaire of 26 items was distributed to all registered nurses (n=2113) in clinical settings within the AHS to elicit responses about their practice of:

- Assessing patients' risk potential for PU development
- Preventing pressure ulcers
- Creating existing ulcers.

For the purpose of this chapter, only the section on assessment will be presented. *Figure 7.1* shows a sample of the questions.

Is an assessment tool, e.g. Norton, Waterlow, Gosnell or other, used on your ward to identify patients 'at risk' of developing pressure ulcer(s)?

Y   N

If yes, which tool do you use? --
How often is the tool used? (When do you assess/reassess?)

If no, when and how do you assess patients 'at risk' of pressure ulcer development? --

Figure 7.1: Assessment

The questionnaire also contained a demographic section and items that explored the overall management process about this area of clinical practice, including documentation.

Content validity of the questionnaire was established by the clinical nurse consultants and clinical nurse specialists who were involved not only in wound management, infection control and PU prevention, but also in the design of the instrument.

Results

The response rate was a disappointing 40% (n=850), and of these only 21% (n=444) of the total 2113 were useable. Many questionnaires were returned in the original bundles with comments such as 'we do not have pressure sores on our ward' or 'not applicable' written on the envelopes.

Nurses, generally, do not use a tool to assess PU risk potential, but rely on a range of practice procedures and risk indicators. Respondents were asked if an assessment tool was used on their ward to identify patients at risk of developing a PU. Less than one-quarter of the respondents (n=95; 21%) indicated that they did use a risk-assessment tool; the most common tool being the Norton (n=75; 79%) (*Table 7.1*).

Table 7.1: Tools used to assess risk of developing a pressure ulcer

Tool(s) used	Number	%
Norton	75	79
Waterlow	12	13
Combination of both	2	2
Other or marked N/A	6	6
Total	*95*	*100*

Respondents were asked when the risk-assessment tool was used. Responses varied widely, and the times ranged between admission of the patient (*n*=37; 39%) to when a PU was noticed (*n*=1; 1%) (*Table 7.2*).

Table 7.2: Timing of risk assessment using a risk-assessment tool

Timing	Number	%
On admission	37	39
As required (PRN)	29	31
Daily	21	22
Weekly	4	4
Post-surgery	1	1
2nd daily	1	1
Very often (commonsense)	1	1
Every time a pressure ulcer is noticed	1	1
Total	*95*	*100*

Most respondents (*n*=349; 79%) did not routinely use a risk-assessment tool in their clinical practice. These respondents were then asked when they assessed their patients for PU risk. Of the 349 respondents, 238 (68%) did not answer the question. It may be assumed that these nurses do not routinely assess their patients for PU risk. The remaining 111 (32%) said they conducted a risk assessment without the use of a tool, and the timing of this assessment generally mirrored the responses given by those who did use a tool (*Table 7.3*).

Table 7.3: Timing of risk assessment without the use of a tool

Timing	Number	%
On admission (O/A)	41	37
As required (PRN)	35	31
Daily	18	16
Each shift	6	5
2nd hourly	3	3
All patients at risk	3	3
2nd daily	1	1
Frequently	1	1
O/A and 2nd hourly when turned	1	1
4th hourly postoperatively	1	1
Ad hoc	1	1
Total	111	100

With regard to how patients were assessed as being at risk if a recognized tool was not used, 166 (48%) nurses responded. Answers were coded as experience (n=94; 57%), if one or more known risk factors were identified, such as immobility, bed rest, age, skin integrity or medical history; or observation (n=72; 43%), if words such as observation, inspection or looking were used (*Table 7.4*).

Table 7.4: How patients were assessed as being at risk if no tool was used

How assessed	Number	%
Experience	94	57
Observation	72	43
Total	166	100

Table 7.5 shows the range of indicators that respondents identified as part of their knowledge base and/or nursing experience to be risk factors for PU development. It can be seen that mobility (or lack of) was the most frequently cited factor that alerted nurses to the patient's risk potential.

Table 7.5: Indicators/risk factors used to assess patients at risk without a recognized tool (coded experience)

Word/phrase used	Frequency
Mobility/bedrest or some equivalent	75
Age and/or elderly	33
Skin integrity/condition of skin	30
Patient weight (including body mass index)	11
Variations on physical condition/frailty	10
Type of operation/surgery/time on operating table	8
Medical/past history	6
Drugs/medications administered	3
Circulation problems	3
Nutritional status	3
Continence/incontinence	2
Mental state	1

N.B. Nurses could identify more than one risk factor

Discussion

The findings support the research conducted by Halfens and Eggink (1995), where a questionnaire was sent to a representative sample of nurses working within Dutch hospitals. Of the 373 questionnaires returned and used for the analysis, 306 nurses (82%) did not use a risk-assessment tool. Similarly, the majority of respondents (*n*=349; 79%) in the present Australian study said they did not use an assessment tool; but of those who did, most used the Norton Scale and a few the Waterlow Scale.

It was evident in the diversity of AHS policies that there is no universally accepted tool or guidelines and no consistent approach to assessment of patients at risk of PU development. Enthusiasm for tools to assess patients varies from strong support to cynical rejection. One respondent commented that 'the last thing nurses want is another b****y form to fill out'!

The first risk-assessment scale was developed in the mid-1950s by Norton (1996), and yet there are no generally agreed upon practice guidelines for this important aspect of PU prevention. The need for user-friendly tools (Hoskins and Ramstadius, 1998) that are both specific and sensitive (Cullum and Clark, 1992) is necessary if nurses are to incorporate assessment into their daily practice; however, it must be conceded that the use of a risk-assessment tool 'does not necessarily ensure accuracy of assessment' (Maylor, 1997).

Whether a recognized tool was used or not, most respondents in the present study indicated that they assessed patients' risk potential on admission, when necessary and/or daily. One commented that a risk-assessment tool was used 'every time a pressure ulcer is noticed'. There is no consistently held view about when an ongoing risk assessment should be undertaken; however, there is some agreement that it should occur at the time of admission. The American-based Agency for Health Care Policy and Research (AHCPR) (Panel for the Prediction and Prevention of Pressure Ulcers in Adults, 1992) recommends the use of a recognized risk-assessment tool on admission to a healthcare facility, and at periodic intervals, for bed and chairbound patients. Ramstadius (1994) is more specific, and recommends that a tool be used on admission, postoperatively and following clinical change.

When a risk-assessment tool is not used, nurses rely on experience and observation to determine whether a patient is at risk of developing a pressure ulcer. The responses for experience were coded if they reflected factors that have been identified in the nursing literature and/or simply as a factor of the respondent's practice experience, as putting a patient at risk of developing a PU. One such well-documented and widely recognized factor is lack of mobility, reflected in the responses of 75 out of 94 responses coded experience.

The next most common risk factor identified by just over a third (n=33) of responses coded experience was increased age or elderly patients. Norton's risk-assessment scale does not include age because the scale was designed for use in an aged-care setting, and perhaps this risk factor was an implicit assumption. Waterlow (1996) suggested that the Norton Scale was not suitable for settings other than aged care and so designed the Waterlow Scale, which rates increasing age alongside lack of mobility as potential risk factors for the development of PUs.

Another surprisingly small number of respondents identified skin integrity or skin condition as a factor to be considered when assessing a patient's risk potential (n=30). Norton (1996) does not mention skin type or condition in her scale, but Ramstadius (1994) includes increased skin temperature in the immobile patient, and Waterlow (1996) includes dry, thin, oedematous and clammy skin as risk factors.

A few respondents (*n*=11) said they assessed body mass index (BMI) to determine risk of PU development, although it is not known how nurses calculated BMI. Piloian (1992) found that BMI had no significance in predicting PU risk. Waterlow (1996) lists both over- and underweight as risk factors, but Norton (1996) lists neither. Hoskins and Ramstadius (1998) maintain that an emaciated patient with full mobility is not at risk, while the same patient with limited mobility is at risk. Although some literature suggests that reduced nutritional intake/poor nutritional status was a risk factor for PU development (Allman et al, 1995; Wiechula, 1997), only a few respondents identified it in this study. Given the potential complexity of undertaking an accurate nutritional assessment (Cullum and Clark, 1992), this is not surprising.

Physical condition/frailty, length of time on the operating table and circulation problems are examples of risk factors that some respondents identified. Clark (1997) found that chronic diseases of the central and peripheral circulation were significant predictive factors for the development of PUs, and the Norton Scale, rather broadly, rates physical (from good to very bad) and mental (from alert to stupor) conditions as risk factors. Waterlow (1998) lists diseases causing tissue malnutrition, neurological deficit, major and orthopaedic surgery, trauma, cytotoxic drugs, high-dose steroids (although high is not defined) and anti-inflammatory drugs as special risk factors. The Ramstadius Scale lists vasoconstriction agents, anaemia, decreased blood supply secondary to disease and pulmonary diseases as risk factors for PU development in the immobile patient (Hoskins and Ramstadius, 1998). Lying for an extended period on hard trolleys or operating tables has been targeted as a particularly serious risk factor for the immobile patient (Waterlow, 1998; Bliss, 1999; Schoonhoven et al, 2002), especially those with a femoral fracture (Versluysen, 1986).

Two respondents in the survey saw incontinence as a contributor to PU development, and this does show up as an independent risk factor in some studies (Woodward, 1998). Brandeis et al (1995) found that a previous history of PU development was strongly associated with the development of other PUs, but this factor was not mentioned by any of the nurses responding to the survey.

Respondents who did not use an assessment tool generally assessed a patient's risk potential using observation or experience. Examples of statements coded observation included:

'Looking at area concerned and deciding whether the patient needs further intervention.'

'Inspection, regular turning and pressure area care.'

'Check skin daily, frequent change of position.'

'Second hourly checking of pressure areas.'

'Visual physical observation as necessary.'

While these statements reflect a basic awareness of the importance of assessing PU risk, they also indicate that a number of nurses assess the patients during routine care procedures such as turns or washes. These nurses did not say how they identified patients that required 'routine care'. Such an approach to assessment could be seen as reactive because the risk may only become evident once the skin has become reddened or broken.

It is clear that risk assessment for PU development is complex, taking into consideration a wide range of potential risk factors. Offering an alternate view, Olshansky (1998) categorized patients as either active (those who have some control in the prevention of PUs) or passive (those who do not). In the latter case, PU development may be related to nursing care. He maintains that PU assessment scales have no accurate predictive value, and the only accurate prediction of risk is the knowledge of the person/nurse who is caring for the patient. The use of alternating-pressure surfaces to relieve pressure for 5-minute intervals has consistently been shown to result in less damage to tissue when compared with tissue subjected to an equivalent amount of constant pressure; this was true even at pressures as high as 240 mmHg for 3 hours (Kosiak, 1961). Therefore, the patient who is provided with an alternating-pressure-air mattress may be less likely to develop a PU than the patient on a static surface, such as a standard hospital mattress.

In summary, less than a quarter of the respondents routinely used a tool to assess patients' risk of developing PUs. Whether a tool was used or not, most nurses indicated that they assessed a patient's risk potential on admission as required (PRN), and/or daily. In general, nurses used their experience and knowledge of risk factors to inform their practice as it relates to the assessment of PU risk. Some, however, relied on routine or regular care procedures as an opportunity to assess risk potential. Overall, the results of this survey indicate quite clearly the lack of consistency with regard to the assessment of patients' risk of developing PUs.

Limitations

Although a sample size of 444 is reasonable, the useable return rate of 21% was disappointing, and generalization of the findings is limited. It is unclear why the response rate was so low. Future surveys may benefit from the identification of one individual in each hospital in an AHS to be responsible for the distribution and collection of surveys. One clinical group involved in this Sydney AHS study that had an 82% response rate used this approach. In addition, a pilot study would have highlighted some of the issues that created difficulties in the analysis of responses.

Recommendations

It is recommended that a PU project group be established within the AHS to undertake several activities:

- Develop clinical practice guidelines/policies based on current nursing research, for the assessment of patients, to identify those at risk
- Evaluate existing tools or, if necessary, develop a tool for the assessment of patients at risk of developing PUs
- The tool should have clearly defined, commonly understood assessment categories, which relate to the aetiology of PU development. It should be objective, reliable, valid, user friendly and have clinical relevance
- Evaluate the tool after implementation.

These findings and others will be reviewed once current practice within the AHS has been identified, and will be used to inform further research. The implementation of an evidence-based approach to practice demands a preliminary understanding of what constitutes current practice.

References

Allman R, Laparde C, Noel L, Walker J, Moorer C, Dear M, Smith C (1986) Pressure sores among hospitalized patients. *Ann Intern Med* **105**: 337–42

Allman RM, Goode PS, Patrick MM, Burst N, Bartolucci AA (1995) Pressure ulcer risk factors among hospitalized patients with activity limitation. *JAMA* **273**(11): 865–70

Bliss M (1999) When are the seeds of postoperative pressure sores sown? — often during surgery. *Br Med J* **319:** 863–4

Boettger JE (1997) Effects of a pressure-reduction mattress and staff education on the incidence of nosocomial pressure ulcers. *J Wound Ostomy Continence Nurs* **24**(1): 19–25

Brandeis GH, Berlowitz DR, Hossain M, Morris JN (1995) Pressure ulcers: the minimum data set and the resident assessment protocol. *Adv Wound Care* **8**(6): 18–25

Callaghan C (1994) Audit changes. *Nurs Times* **90**(35): 69–70, 74

Clark M (1997) Master class: pressure sore treatment, evidence of effectiveness. *J Wound Care* **6**(8): 400–2

Crow R (1988) The challenge of pressure sores. *Nurs Times* **84**(38): 68–73

Cullum N, Clark M (1992) Intrinsic factors associated with pressure sores in elderly people. *J Adv Nurs* **17**: 427–431

Curry, K, Casady L (1992) The relationship between extended periods of immobility and decubitus ulcer formation in the acutely spinal cord-injured individual. *J Neurosci Nurs* **24**(4): 185–9

Dimond B (1994) Pressure sores: a case to answer. *Br J Nurs* **3**(14): 721–7

Exton-Smith AN (1987) The patients not for turning. *Nurs Times* **83**(42): 42–4

Exton-Smith AN, Sherwin RW (1961) The prevention of pressure sores: significance of spontaneous bodily movements. *Lancet* **2**: 1124–6

Fletcher RJ (1997) Master class: pressure sore treatment. *J Wound Care* **6**(8): 398–9

Halfens R, Eggink M (1995) Knowledge, beliefs and use of nursing methods in preventing pressure sores in Dutch hospitals. *Int J Nurs Stud* **35**: 16–26

Hawthorn PJ, Nyquist R (1988) The incidence of pressure sores amongst a group of elderly patients with fractured neck of femur. *CARE — Science and Practice* **6**(13): 3–17

Hibbs P (1982) Pressure sores: a system of prevention. *Nurs Mirror* 155: 1311–13

Hoskins A, Ramstadius B (1998) Risk assessment for pressure sores: a comparison of two tools. *Primary Intention* **6**(4): 160–7

Jiricka MK, Ryan P, Carvalho MA, Bukvich J (1995) Pressure ulcer risk factors in an ICU population. *Am J Crit Care* **4**(5): 361–7

Klei M, MacLellan L, MacLellan D (1997) Bottoms up: avoiding the horrors of pressure ulcers. *Veterans' Health* **20**: 24–7

Kosiak M (1961) Etiology of decubitus ulcers. *Arch Phys Med Rehab* **42**(January): 19–29

Lockyer-Stevens N (1993) The use of water-filled gloves to prevent the formation of decubitus ulcers on heels. *J Wound Care* **2**(5): 282–5

Maylor ME (1997) Knowledge base and use in the management of pressure sores. *J Wound Care* **6**(5): 244–7

Norton D (1996) Calculating the risk: reflections on the Norton Scale. *Adv Wound Care* **9**(6): 38–43

Olshansky K (1998) Pressure ulcer risk assessment scales: the missing link, a commentary. *Adv Wound Care* **7**(3): 64–8

Panel for the Prediction and Prevention of Pressure Ulcers in Adults (1992) *Pressure Ulcers in Adults: Prediction and Prevention Clinical Practice*

Guideline, Number 3. AHCPR Publication No 92-0047. Agency for Health Care Policy and Research, Public Health Service, US Department of Health and Human Services, Rockville, MD, USA

Pearson A (1997) New survey puts pressure on health's running sore. *Australian Health and Aged Care Journal* **20:** 97–9

Piloian B (1992) Defining characteristics of the nursing diagnosis 'high risk for impaired skin integrity'. *Decubitus* **5**(5): 32–47

Quickfall J, Shields D (1998) Peak performance. *Nurs Times* **94**(7): 74–7

Ramstadius B (1994) *In-Depth Semistructured Tape-Recorded Interview by Sharp CA*. Wollongong Hospital, Wollongong, New South Wales, Australia

Schoonhoven L, Defloor T, Grypdonck MHF (2002) Incidence of pressure ulcers due to surgery. *J Clin Nurs* **11**(4): 479–87

Sharp C, Burr G, Broadbent M, Cummins M, Casey H, Merriman A (2000) Pressure ulcer prevention and care: a survey of current practice. *J Qual Clin Pract* **20:** 150–7

Versluysen M (1986) How elderly patients with femoral fracture develop pressure sores in hospital. *Br Med J* **292:** 1311–13

Waterlow JA (1996) Pressure sore risk assessment: a pressure sore risk scale for use with older people. *Prof Nurse* **11**(11): 713

Waterlow J (1998) The history and use of the Waterlow card. *Nurs Times* **94**(7): 63–7

Whittle H, Fletcher C, Hoskin A, Campbell K (1996) Nursing management of pressure ulcers using a hydrogel dressing protocol: four case studies. *Rehabil Nurs* **21**(5): 239–42

Wiechula R (1997) *Pressure Sores, Part 1: Prevention of Pressure Related Damage*. Best Practice: Evidence-Based Practice Information Sheets for Health Professionals. Blackwell Science Asia, Carlton, Australia

Woodward M (1998) Risk factors: do they withstand pressure? Unpublished paper presented at The Second Australian Wound Management Association Conference, Brisbane, 18–21 March

Young C (1997) What cost a pressure ulcer? *Primary Intention* **5**(4): 24–5, 28–31

Zernicke W (1997) Heel pressure-relieving devices: how effective are they? *Aust J Adv Nurs* **14**(4): 12–9

Chapter 8

Pressure ulcer benchmarking within a primary care setting

Naomi Burbridge, Sarah Kiernan

Patient-focused benchmarking was initially launched by the Department of Health. This chapter examines how the tissue viability service of Camden and Islington primary care trusts implemented the pressure ulcer benchmarking process within the nursing teams of these trusts. This was achieved by: agreeing best practice through examination of local and national guidelines; developing a suitable audit tool for nursing teams to assess their clinical areas against this best practice; nursing teams producing core action plans to facilitate movement towards best practice; disseminating results; and reauditing. The results of the audits carried out in October 2003 and February 2004 are presented. A plan for future work is described including the involvement of other members of the multidisciplinary team and the Patient Advice Liaison Service, and linking pressure ulcer benchmarking to the benchmarks of communication, privacy and dignity, and record keeping.

The Department of Health's (DoH, 2001) patient-focused benchmarks document *Essence of Care* was launched as a framework for standardizing key fundamental aspects of care. The aim was to provide a toolkit for improving the quality of care and services offered to patients, placing the process firmly within the clinical governance agenda. Clinicians and managers can use the tool to measure current practice and service against set national standards, plan steps to improve areas found to be short of the ideal and re-evaluate. One of the benchmarks relates to pressure ulcers and is aimed at preventing skin breakdown. It contains nine factors with associated best practice statements

Table 8.1: Benchmarks for pressure ulcers	
Factor	**Statement (benchmark) of best practice**
1. Screening and assessment	For all patients identified as 'at risk', screening should progress to further assessment
2. Who undertakes assessment	Patients are assessed by assessors who have the required specific knowledge and expertise and have ongoing updating
3. Informing patients and carers	Patients and/or carers have ongoing access to information and have the opportunity to discuss this and its relevance to their individual needs
4. Individualized plan for prevention and treatment	Individualized documented plan agreed with the multidisciplinary team in partnership with patients and/or carers, with evidence of ongoing reassessment
5. Repositioning	The patient's need for repositioning has been assessed, documented, met and evaluated with evidence of ongoing reassessment
6. Redistributing support surfaces	Patients at risk of developing pressure ulcers are cared for on pressure-redistributing support surfaces that meet individual needs, including comfort
7. Availability of resources/ equipment	Patients have all the equipment they require to meet their individual needs
8. Implementation of individualized plan	The plan is fully implemented in partnership with the multidisciplinary team, patients and/or carers
9. Evaluation of interventions by a registered practitioner	An evaluation that incorporates patients and/or carers' participation in forward planning is documented

From DoH (2001)

(*Table 8.1*). This chapter examines how the tissue viability service (TVS) in Islington and Camden primary care trusts (PCTs) began the process of implementing the benchmark for pressure ulcers.

Following publication of the *Essence of Care* document (DoH, 2001), the TVS in Islington and Camden PCTs began the process of pressure ulcer benchmarking with the nursing staff in the following areas: district nursing services; older people's service and mental health care of older people's wards at St Pancras Hospital; and local nursing homes. It was acknowledged that pressure ulcer prevention and management was an area of relevance to other healthcare professionals in the trusts, but the decision was made to invite them later when the process was clearly understood and established by the nursing staff.

The first step was to establish a group to lead implementation at clinical level. To ensure that the process was seen as a priority, it was considered vital that senior clinical staff, such as team leaders, matrons, link nurses and clinical governance managers, were involved from the beginning, and so they were invited to form the initial pressure ulcer benchmarking group. Involving nurses from across a variety of clinical settings enabled wide dissemination of the process and allowed broad comparison and sharing of good practice.

To update the members of the group with the national and local standards relating to pressure ulcer prevention and management, the following documents were reviewed at the first meeting: *Essence of Care* (DoH, 2001), National Institute for Clinical Excellence (NICE, 2001a) guidelines, Royal College of Nursing (RCN, 2001) guidelines and local guidelines (Kiernan, 2000). These documents were examined to see how evidence of achieving best practice statements could be supported. Copies can now be found in all clinical areas.

To measure how current practice related to the benchmarks (see *Table 8.1*), the TVS adopted an audit tool that had been developed, with PCT representation, at a local acute hospital trust. The tool contained sections requiring examination of documentation, observation of practice, and questions to staff about pressure ulcer prevention and management practice.

The first audit of clinical areas took place in May 2003 and involved an external and internal scorer analyzing a sample of 10 patients. The scorers then had to agree on a score from 'A' (best practice) to 'E' (worst practice) (DoH, 2001) for each factor. The forms were sent to the TVS for analysis.

Feedback on the process took place in the form of written anonymous evaluation forms and discussion at the next meeting. The following problems were identified:

- The tool was complex, long and time consuming, leading to incomplete forms

- Difficulty formulating action plans to assist movement towards best practice
- Difficulty allocating a benchmark, as the descriptors between 'A' and 'E' did not have clear parameters
- Difficulty arranging mutually convenient times with an external scorer
- Questions repeated in different sections
- District nurses needed extra time to look at patients' home and base notes.

As a result of the feedback, which coincided with the re-formatting of the original benchmarks by the Modernisation Agency (2003), the TVS changed the audit tool and presented it to the benchmarking group for agreement.

In the revised audit tool the number of questions were significantly reduced and were set out using the nursing process framework, as this was a format with which everyone was familiar. Questions had either a 'yes' or 'no' answer. Only if all the answers to the questions were 'yes' would the best practice benchmarks be reached. If any question was answered 'no', then an action plan needed to be drawn up to facilitate movement towards best practice. The teams were required to audit five patients, and no external auditor was required. These changes were made to speed the audit process and to show that the nurses were trusted to measure accurately current practice in their own teams.

During October 2003 and February 2004 respectively, a total of 35 teams were invited to audit five patients each who had, or were at risk of, pressure ulceration, giving a possible total of 175 audits. In October 2003, 55 (31.4%) forms were returned from 13 areas, and 54 (30.8%) from 12 areas for February 2004. Not all teams audited five patients. This was found to be because some members of the benchmarking group did not attend the audit planning meetings, some members left and replacements had not been allocated and some teams experienced increase in workload during these times. Discussion and written evaluation at this time in relation to the new tool stated that:

- Instructions were easier to follow
- It was easier not to have to allocate a score for each benchmark
- Action planning was easier
- The process was less time consuming, taking an average of 15 minutes to complete per patient.

Tables 8.2–8.6 provide a summary of the responses to the questions asked in these audits. No direct comparison for individual teams is provided, as in some cases different teams responded on each audit. It is noted that this will affect the results, as different teams will have different practices. The responsibility was for the individual teams to compare their own results on different audits.

Audit results

Assessment

In February 2004, all patients had received a risk assessment using an appropriate tool; a registered nurse did not sign 3.6% of these. There was a large increase of 53.9% from October 2003 in the number of patients who had

Question	Oct '03	Feb '04	Progress ↑↓
1. Does the patient have a Norton/ Walsall score?	100.0	100.0	–
2a. Was the Norton/Walsall score dated?	96.3	98.2	1.9↑
2b. Was the Norton/Walsall score timed?	40.7	94.6	53.9↑
2c. Was the Norton/Walsall signed by a RN?	92.6	96.4	3.8↑
3. Was the risk assessment completed within 2 hours of admission (hospital) or on the first visit (community)?	90.7	91.0	0.3↑
4. Has continence been assessed?	90.7	92.8	2.1↑
5. Has a nutritional assessment been recorded (including weight)?	81.5	83.6	2.1↑
6. Has a moving and handling assessment been recorded?	90.7	89.1	1.6↓

Table 8.2: Percentage of adults responding 'yes' to questions about assessment of patients with or 'at risk' of pressure ulceration

↑=increase between October 2003 and February 2004; ↓=decrease between October 2003 and February 2004; –=no change in percentage between October 2003 and February 2004; RN=registered nurse

the assessment timed, allowing the wards to assess whether it had been completed within 2 hours of admission (in line with local guidelines) and meeting record-keeping standards, the total percentage of timed assessments being 94.6% in February 2004. Of these assessments, 91% were completed within the necessary timeframe (*Table 8.2*).

Planning

In February 2004, 98.2% of patients had a plan of care (*Table 8.3*). There was an increase in the inclusion of the following in the plan: details of skin

Table 8.3: Percentage of adults responding 'yes' to questions about planning of care for patients with or 'at risk' of pressure ulceration			
Question	**Oct '03**	**Feb '04**	**Progress↑↓**
7. Does the patient have a care plan?	96.3	98 2	1.9↑
8a. Does the plan include a repositioning regimen?	64.1	47.3	16.8↓
8b. Does the plan include details of skin assessment (in line with guideline)?	68.5	78.2	9.7↑
8c. Does the plan include identification of specifc risks?	81.5	87.3	5.8↑
8d. Does the plan include name of equipment in use?	79.6	80.0	0.4↑
8e. Does the plan include if a dynamic system is used, and are the details of the mattress settings documented?	63.0	81.8	18 8↑
8f. Does the plan include date equipment installed?	75.9	67.3	8.6↓
8h. Does the plan include signature of RN?	81.5	81.8	0.3↑
9. Is a pressure ulcer present? (If no go to Q12)	44.4	72.8	28.4↑

↑=increase between October 2003 and February 2004; ↓=decrease between October 2003 and February 2004; –=no change in percentage between October 2003 and February 2004; RN=registered nurse

assessment, identification of specific risks, name of equipment in use and settings on dynamic system (if used). There was, however, a 16.8% decrease in the number of patients who had a repositioning regimen. This negative change in repositioning was unexpected given discussions about this at *Essence of Care* meetings and the presentation and dissemination of different means of recording such regimens. It may reflect a change in the education level of the nurses, as it had been explained to them that the repositioning regimens needed to be individualized and based on skin inspection. Therefore, more nurses may have ticked 'No' on the audit, because there was no evidence that the provided regimen was specific for that patient.

There was also a negative change (8.6%) in the number of patients having the date equipment was installed recorded. This could be related to the number of patients audited requiring equipment being larger than in the last audit. This explanation is supported by the fact that more patients audited had a pressure ulcer present in the February audit (increase of 28.4%).

Patient care

In relation to the assessment and planning of care for these pressure ulcers, every patient with an ulcer had a wound assessment chart, and there was an increase of 8.3% in the number of patients who had their ulcer staged, bringing the total to 93.4%. In the wound care plans, the location of the ulcer was documented for all patients, as was the dressing selection and frequency of dressing change. The documentation of the patients' pain level increased by 28.4% to 86.7%, and the rationale for dressing choice increased by 15.9%, giving a total inclusion of 86.7% (*Table 8.4*).

Implementation

In February 2004, 98.2% of patients had documentation that the care that was planned for them was implemented, and all of these entries were signed and dated by a trained member of staff. There was a 16.1% decrease in patient and carer involvement. This increase in a lack of patient and carer involvement is also seen when evaluating care.

Various explanations can be put forward for this: it could be owing to the mental health of the patients being audited, preventing them from understanding new information at that time; or that the patient is an inpatient with no visiting family/carer. However, it could also reflect a lack of

Table 8.4: Percentage of adults responding 'yes' to questions about care of patients with pressure ulceration

Question	Oct '03	Feb '04	Progress↑↓
10a. Is there documentation of stage of ulcer?	79.2	93.4	14.2↑
10b. Is there documentation of wound assessment chart?	91.7	100.0	8.3↑
10c. Is there documentation of wound reassessment date?	100 0	93 4	6.6↓
10d. Is there documentation of tracing or photograph?	58.3	67.0	8.7↑
11a. Does the care plan contain the details of location of ulcer?	100.0	100.0	–
11b. Does the care plan contain the details of pain level?	58. 3	86.7	28.4↑
11c. Does the care plan contain the details of dressing selection?	100.0	100.0	–
11d. Does the care plan contain the details of frequency of dressing change?	95.3	100.0	4.7%↑
11e. Does the care plan contain the details of rationale for choice of dressing?	70.8	86.7	15.9
11f. Does the care plan contain the details of reassessment date?	95.3	100.0	4.7↑

↑=increase between October 2003 and February 2004; ↓=decrease between October 2003 and February 2004; –=no change in percentage between October 2003 and February 2004

collaborative working with social services within the community setting. Multidisciplinary team involvement took place an appropriate 94.6% of the time.

In February 2004, 83.6% of staff providing patient care had received ongoing training in pressure ulcer prevention and management. There was a decrease of 12.6% from October 2003 in the number of staff receiving ongoing training for equipment. This could be related to the fact that the last equipment

Table 8.5: Percentage of adults responding 'yes' to questions about implementation of care for patients with or 'at risk' of pressure ulceration

Question	Oct '03	Feb '04	Progress↑↓
12. Is the individualized plan being implemented?	96.3	98.2	1.9↑
13. Is variance from the plan documented?	92.6	81.8	10.8↓
14. Is there evidence of patient/ carer involvement?	85.2	69.1	16.1↓
15. Is there evidence of MDT referral/ involvement as necessary?	94.4	94.6	0.2↑
16. Are all entries signed and dated by trained staff member?	94.4	100.0	5.6↑
17a. Have all the staff members providing care to this patient received ongoing training in pressure ulcer prevention and management?	81.5	83.6	2.1↑
17b. Have all the staff members providing care to this patient received ongoing training in equipment?	94.4	81.8	12.6↓
18. Has the patient been given a pressure ulcer information booklet?	40.7	69.1	28.4↑
19. Is there evidence that the leaflet has been discussed with the patient?	46.3	52.8	6.5↑
20. Does the patient have all the equipment required to implement care, e.g. moving and handling, redistribution support surface and electric profile bed?	96.3	96.4	0.1↑
21. Does equipment arrive when requested?	96.3	96.4	0.1%↑
22. Is there evidence that the patient has been made aware of how to use the equipment safely and what to do in the event of breakdown?	85.2	87.3	2.1%↑
23a. In relation to equipment, are there procedures in place and followed for repair?	94.4	100.0	5.6%↑
23b. In relation to equipment, are there procedures in place and followed for maintenance?	94.4	100.0	5.6%↑
23c. In relation to equipment, are there procedures in place and followed for infection control?	90.7	92.7	2.0%↑

↑=increase between October 2003 and February 2004; ↓=decrease between October 2003 and February 2004; –=no change in percentage between October 2003 and February 2004; MDT=multidisciplinary team

exhibition run by the trusts was in November 2002, so on the date of the first audit nursing staff would have had an update in the last year, but at the second audit this would then be out of date. In February 2004, 69.1% of patients received a pressure ulcer information leaflet, an increase of 28.4%.

All the equipment required to implement care was provided for 96.4% of patients and this arrived within the time requested 96.4% of the time (*Table 8.5*).

Table 8.6: Percentage of adults responding 'yes' to questions about evaluation of care for patients with or 'at risk' of pressure ulceration

Question	Oct '03	Feb '04	Progress↑↓
24. Is there evidence that actions have been evaluated and is reassessment in line with guideline?	88.9	92.7	3.8↑
25. Is there evidence of patient/carer involvement in evaluating outcomes?	81.5	69.1	12.4↓

↑=increase between October 2003 and February 2004; ↓=decrease between October 2003 and February 2004; –=no change in percentage between October 2003 and February 2004

Evaluation

Care was evaluated in line with guidelines for 92.7% of patients, an increase of 3.8%. However, patient and carer involvement with this evaluation decreased by 12.4%, as discussed above (*Table 8.6*).

Action planning

Following both audits, comparison group meetings were held to share and compare best practice and develop action plans to facilitate movement towards the best practice benchmarks. Analysis of the action plans highlighted two points:

■ There were common areas where action planning needed to take place
■ Some teams were only action planning for the patient they had audited,

rather than taking a more global perspective of their team and looking at ways they could achieve the best practice benchmark for all the patients under their care.

This led to the development of some 'core action plans' by the comparison group and TVS in order to guide other members in the format that the action plans should take, share ideas on how best practice could be reached and to save everyone time. These were then disseminated to all teams.

These action plans introduced a number of changes to nursing practice including:

- Allocating responsibility to a staff member to order the booklet *Working Together to Prevent Pressure Ulcers: a Guide for Patients and Carers* (NICE, 2001b), to ensure a continuous stock. Following a first assessment, other team members are then asked to follow up and check that the booklet has been given and read by the patient, and his/her understanding has been assessed
- Admission packs were to be made up containing all the necessary assessments required for determining if a patient is at risk of pressure ulceration and to help plan the necessary steps to reduce this risk. Other team members were then allocated responsibility to check these had all been completed, thus involving more junior staff members in the process
- A template-training chart was disseminated to allow other staff members to identify the competency of their colleagues when allocating work. The formal dissemination of knowledge gained from study days, which not all members could attend because of staffing shortages, was encouraged
- Repositioning charts were disseminated to allow the recording of advised and actual repositioning regimens. These were to be used by district nurses and social services. Turning clocks were also introduced to group members and implemented as prompts for patients and their carers. Turning clocks are paper circles surrounded by numbers, which staff can use to indicate at what time and into which position the patient has agreed to be moved
- A template of a pressure ulcer prevention care plan was provided as a prompt for nurses to use
- Comparison group members were provided with diary-sized copies of the Stirling Pressure Ulcer Severity Scale (Reid and Morrison, 1994) to allow accurate descriptions of pressure ulcers. Other staff members were encouraged to check staging on subsequent visits and to discuss this at team meetings to try and reduce reliability problems in wound assessment.

Comparison group evaluation

In February 2004, an evaluation of the process so far took place in the form of a questionnaire — this presented statements about the benchmarking that participants had to rate using a five-point scale from 'strongly disagree' to 'strongly agree'. This was sent to all members of the comparison group who had completed an audit in February 2004 or October 2003. Eighteen evaluations were sent and 15 were returned, giving a response rate of 83.3%.

Everyone agreed that attendance at the *Essence of Care* meetings had improved their knowledge of current policy requirements for the care of patients, with or at risk of pressure ulceration. They also all agreed that the auditing of their area of work against standards had been helpful in showing where changes needed to take place.

Twelve respondents agreed that changes have taken place as a result of increased knowledge and action planning, but three respondents were unsure. The reason for people being unsure could be because of different people carrying out the audits and staff turnover preventing them being able to identify and evaluate the effects of the action planning. Of those who said that changes had taken place, these included: giving patients information through booklets and discussion, including a repositioning regimen in the plan of care and keeping the care plan updated; documenting times of risk assessment; and completing wound assessment charts. Constraints made it difficult to implement changes for seven of respondents — these included: time constraints, shortage of staff, staff lacking education and not following instructions and a lack of motivation. To help them implement the action plans they proposed the following: increasing the number of staff on wards, teamwork, staff education and opportunity to feed back to colleagues.

Respondents also commented that they found the outcomes of the benchmarking positive and that it helped to reinforce to the team members all the work that they were doing under difficult staffing conditions.

Challenges to implementation

The challenges encountered in this trust are similar to those noted by Chambers and Jolly (2002), including:

- 'Lack of resources' — difficulties occurred in maintaining continuity in attendance of comparison group members because of heavy workloads

and staff shortages. This led to one trust allocating two nurses to attend as representatives and feed back to their colleagues
- 'People assuming responsibility' — although it is acknowledged that each team should be responsible for ensuring that pressure ulcer benchmarking continues regularly, it could be suggested that the continued involvement of the TVS is required to lead and collate the process
- 'Moving from enthusiasm to commitment' — as all the other benchmarks outlined in *Essence of Care* also needed implementation, it was soon easy to observe that teams were getting bogged down in meetings and paper-work. This meant that after the benchmarking regimen had been estab-lished, meetings were reduced from monthly to quarterly.

Dissemination

Dissemination has taken place via the trusts' strategic planning group for *Essence of Care*, encouraging comparison group members to discuss issues raised at meetings with their team and through presentation at a North Central Sector Strategic Health Authority event.

Future plans

When the comparison group was asked how they wanted to see *Essence of Care* moving forward, they responded:

- Seeking patients' and families' views on the way care is delivered
- Expanding tools for auditing best practice to incorporate more aspects
- Involvement/training with other disciplines
- Incorporating *Essence of Care* benchmarks into local tissue viability guidelines.

This was encouraging to read, as this is where the TVS had planned to take the agenda forward.

A new tool is being developed to audit different factors, including those from the privacy and dignity, communication and record-keeping benchmark, in relation to pressure area care. During the last comparison group meeting, it was discussed how these benchmarks relate to the pressure ulcer benchmark and how these could be incorporated into the audit tool to show how areas of these benchmarks are being met.

Other concurrent work to facilitate movement towards the best practice benchmarks by the TVS has included:

- Improving access to pressure ulcer prevention study days by allowing staff from Barnet, Haringey, Islington and Camden to attend study days held by any of these trusts
- Meetings with those involved in integrated community equipment store to improve access to equipment required in pressure ulcer-prevention strategies
- Dissemination of local (Kiernan, 2000) and NICE (2001b, 2003) guidelines on pressure ulcer prevention. The local guidelines are currently under review, and it is planned that they will be relaunched this year
- A pressure ulcer-prevention programme has been run in older people services, and the link nurse system has been reinitiated to allow senior staff members to educate other members of the nursing team. There are plans to roll this out to the other nurses who form the comparison group
- Multidisciplinary team meetings were started in June 2004, including occupational therapists, physiotherapists and therapists from the wheelchair centre, to examine their contribution to the benchmarks
- As a result of an observed rise in advice sought from nursing homes around pressure ulcer management from the TVS, a two-part nursing home pressure ulcer prevention study day was run in November 2003 and January 2004 specifically to target needs of nursing homes
- There are plans to involve the Patient Advice and Liaison Service in future evaluations.

Conclusion

The implementation of benchmarking for pressure ulcers is now firmly established and improvements in practice are beginning to be seen. After further audits, it will become clearer what are the direct effects of the process on clinical practice and patient care. The next step will be to compare and share practice with the surrounding acute and community trusts to gain a greater comparison field. The benchmarking process has not been used in isolation; educational outreach has been run concurrently with the audit and feedback process to help practitioners apply knowledge and available research and guidelines to practice.

References

Chambers N, Jolly A (2002) Essence of Care: making a difference. *Nurs Stand* **17**(11): 40–4

Department of Health (2001) *Essence of Care: Patient-focused Benchmarking for Health Care Practitioners.* DoH, London

Kiernan S (2000) *Local Guidelines for the Prevention and Management of Pressure Ulcers.* Camden and Islington Community Health Services NHS Trust, London

Modernisation Agency (2003) *Essence of Care: Patient-focused Benchmarks for Clinical Governance.* DoH, London

National Institute for Clinical Excellence (NICE) (2001a) *Pressure Ulcer Risk Assessment and Prevention.* NICE, London

NICE (2001b) *Working Together to Prevent Pressure Ulcers: a Guide for Patients and Their Carers.* NICE, London

NICE (2003) *Pressure Ulcer Prevention: Pressure Ulcer Risk Assessment and Prevention, Including the Use of Pressure Relieving Devices (Beds, Mattresses and Overlays) for the Prevention of Pressure Ulcers in Primary and Secondary Care.* NICE, London

Reid J, Morrison M (1994) Towards a consensus: classification of pressure sore. *J Wound Care* **3**: 157–60

Royal College of Nursing (2001) *Clinical Practice Guidelines: Pressure Ulcer Risk Assessment and Prevention.* RCN, London

Chapter 9

A static-led approach to pressure ulcers: an evaluation after 3 years

Jane James

Pressure damage has high cost implications to the patient and care providers. The choice of appropriate equipment to help in the prevention of tissue damage is hampered by extensive choice and little guidance on the most effective product to use. The static-led approach was introduced into Carmarthenshire NHS Trust 3 years ago. This approach simplified the choice of equipment, improving the appropriate usage and reducing expenditure. This chapter evaluates the approach 3 years after its introduction to determine if the benefits to the patient and the organization still apply.

Selecting equipment for pressure damage prevention is complex and challenging. Despite recent recommendations from the National Institute for Clinical Excellence (NICE) relating to pressure-relieving equipment (NICE, 2003), there still appears to be little evidence to support individual pieces of equipment.

Three years ago in an acute general hospital in the author's trust, effective coordination and management of pressure-damage prevention was not evident. This resulted in pressure-reducing equipment being procured at ward level with decisions being based on financial and individual preferences. The equipment was not standardized and remained at ward level with no rationale for its use, often being stored in bathrooms or under patients who were mobile and independent. Servicing of the equipment was reactionary and often led to equipment failure in periods of high demand. As a result, escalating rental costs of over £200 000 per year and a pressure-ulcer prevalence rate of 30% became a driving force to coordinate and rationalize the management of pressure-reducing equipment.

In response to this, a project team of clinical, managerial, procurement and finance representatives was set up to establish the resource requirements of the hospital by evaluating the equipment need in clinical practice. A prerequisite was to establish a programme of care within the constraints of current expenditure. The group decided to adopt a static-led approach (Thomas and James, 2002).

The static-led approach

The fundamental principle of a static-led approach is to provide an environment in which pressure ulcers do not develop or existing pressure ulcers improve. However, ensuring that the patient is being nursed on an appropriate mattress for his/her need was not always being achieved. It has been suggested that the problem of pressure ulcer development could potentially be resolved through the provision of appropriate pressure-reducing equipment to those individuals at risk (Maylor, 2001).

In order to improve appropriate use of equipment, the static-led approach ensured simplicity in equipment choice. All patients would be nursed on a standardized, pressure-redistributing foam mattress (MSS Softform), except those who were assessed through the combined use of a risk-assessment tool and clinical judgment to be at high risk of developing pressure damage. These patients would be nursed on a dynamic mattress system suitable for their level of need (Cairwave, Pegasus Ltd, Hampshire). It was recognized that suitable pressure- reducing surfaces (if required) should be used when the patient is seated, and an important part of the approach was ensuring that appropriate cushions were allocated to patients at any level of risk of developing pressure damage (Collins, 2004).

It is accepted by the author that there appears to be much negativity when writing about risk-assessment tools. However, some positive attributes are that by standardizing the assessment process of patients and prompting nurses by highlighting the risk factors, they can create a framework on which appropriate care is provided. It has been said that the introduction of risk-assessment tools in conjunction with the establishment of education programmes and protocols may reduce the incidence of pressure ulcers (McGough, 1999), and it is generally accepted that they will help to identify the next care intervention (Collier, 2001). The use of scales alone to assess patient risk cannot be supported on the basis of current evidence, and while a risk-assessment tool can be an important part in an overall pressure ulcer prevention strategy, it should be an aid to clinical judgment and not a substitute for it (Scott, 2000).

As part of a 7-year managed programme in the author's trust, all foam mattresses were replaced, gel cushions were procured and dynamic mattresses were leased, in which a servicing and repair contract was also included. The benefits of the static-led approach are listed in *Table 9.1*.

Table 9.1: Benefits of a static-led approach

- Effective equipment selection from a two-system approach increased appropriate usage by simplifying mattress choice

- A high level of protection was given to all patients admitted to hospital because all beds had a redistribution foam mattress, which offers a high level of protection against pressure damage

- Significant reduction in the number of dynamic mattresses as a result of using the foam mattress for all patients, apart from those assessed to be at high risk of pressure damage

- Reduced costs as a result of the reduction in the number of dynamic mattress systems

- Positive staff satisfaction survey (Thomas and James, 2002)

- Equipment available at point of need. This means that the gap between identified need and the appropriate therapy for the patient is reduced, and also a reduction in the time wasted by staff in hiring or phoning other clinical areas for equipment allows more time to concentrate on patient care

- Reduced prevalence rate as a result of more patients being nursed on the appropriate mattress for their level of need

The dynamic systems are on a 7-year leasing contract and all static systems were purchased with a rolling replacement programme set up. To fully implement, manage and develop the programme, a tissue viability nurse (TVN) was appointed. Mattresses were located in a centralized store and allocated to wards as per individual patient need. A support worker was appointed to facilitate the process. This resulted in a more manageable and cost-effective system.

In line with NICE (2001) guidelines, initial risk assessment was within 6 hours of admission, and a core care plan was introduced to facilitate ongoing assessment of patient risk status, promote the appropriate allocation of systems and provide an audit trail. This 7-year programme of care, inclusive of the appointment of the TVN and support worker, was achieved within current expenditure and included significant cost savings.

Three years later

The initial benefits of the managed system were evident; however, could these benefits be maintained 3 years after the introduction of the static-led approach?

The amalgamation with a neighbouring hospital had seen an increase of beds to nearly 700, and it was decided to standardize the approach across the trust. All dynamic mattresses, apart from those that offered a high level of support, were removed from the second hospital and a variety of foam mattresses were replaced with MSS Softform. Cushions were replaced and documentation was standardized.

Training and education is ongoing throughout the whole trust in all the clinical and operational aspects of pressure damage prevention.

Documentation

Assessment of the patient's risk status using clinical judgment and a formal tool (*Figure 9.1*) were seen as playing a key role in the success of the static-led approach.

Patients at risk are assessed daily and 'stepped up or down' from the dynamic mattresses depending on their clinical condition (in accordance with local policy). Initially, there was no place in the nursing documentation to record the patient's risk score and compliance identified on audit was poor, with less than 40% of patients having an up-to-date assessment. The introduction of a standardized care plan in line with the NICE (2003) guidelines allows for the risk assessment to be accessible to all members of the interdisciplinary team (see *Figure 9.1*). It has also increased the number of patients having an up-to-date assessment to 85%.

Name of Patient

Problem/need:

PSPS	<6	☐
PSPS	6–9	☐
PSPS	10–11	☐
PSPS	12–16	☐

Objective:

Preventive ☐

— To reduce/relieve pressure

— To maintain skin integrity

— To monitor effects of prevention measure

Treatment ☐

— To relieve pressure

— To promote healing

— To monitor effects of treatment and nursing intervention

Plan of care

Has the plan of care been discussed and agreed with patient or relative? Yes ☐   No ☐

If no, specify reason:

Prevention ☐   Healing ☐

PSPS 6

Re-assess as condition changes

PSPS 6–9

1) Pressure-reducing foam mattress

2) Pressure reducing cushion   Type: _____

3) Regular repositioning   Frequency: Minimum 2 hourly

4) Encourage independent movement by the client

PSPS 10–11

1) Pressure-reducing foam mattress

2) Pressure reducing/relieving cushion   Type: _____

3) Regular repositioning   Frequency: Minimum 2 hourly

4) Encourage independent movement by the client

PSPS 12–16

1) Cairwave

2) Pressure reducing/relieving cushion

Daycare ☐   Pro-Active ☐   Floteck Solution ☐

3) If pressure ulcer present initiate wound assessment form

Signature: _____   *Date:* _____

Please see overleaf

PSPS ABOVE 6: **Daily assessment**
PSPS BELOW 6: **Weekly assessment or as condition changes**

Date	PSPS	Comment	Signature

Figure 9.1: Pressure Sore Prediction Score (PSPS) assessment tool
From Lothian (1989)

Mattress selection

Initially there was a concern that the static mattresses would be compromised by the need for frequent movement between wards and the equipment library. However, the MSS Softform mattresses have been audited annually and, in agreement with Gray et al (1998), have continued to perform well. There has been no evidence of loss of function of the foam. Replacement covers and inserts have been unremarkable and within anticipated budget allowances of £1000 per annum.

The dynamic mattresses that are on a lease agreement have ensured a constant supply of appropriate equipment for those patients at high risk of pressure damage. An agreed rental pool of five mattresses allows immediate access if all leased systems are in use, without the delivery time and costs normally incurred.

An original budget of £10 000 per annum was allocated in the programme for anticipated rental costs. However, over the past year the actual rental spend was less than £1500 for the two hospital sites combined.

Centralized equipment library

An equipment library was opened in the second hospital and a support worker employed to facilitate this and provide support in the delivery and installation of the equipment. Owing to the success in reducing the amount of equipment, it was decided to extend both libraries to include infusion devices. Since opening, the libraries have been met with a positive response from nursing, portering and medical electronics staff. The equipment has been well used and kept stored in a clean condition, and is readily available at the point of need.

Equipment needing routine servicing can be sought using an electronic tracking system, which has proved to be effective in saving both time and resources. Equipment is selected from a request form (*Figure 9.2*), which initiates the first stage of the tracking, and decontamination forms returned with the equipment end the process.

The libraries have facilitated a reduction in the amount of infusion devices needed, which has resulted in further cost savings for the trust.

Ward		Patient's ID No.	
Date		Signature (staff requesting equipment)	
Time			

Item requested

Infusion device
(Please tick appropriate box)

PPH
Graseby 500 volumetric pump (wards 5 and 6 only)
Baxter 6201/6200 volumetric pump (wards 1, 2, 3, 4, 7 and 8 only)
Alaris (IVAC) P2000 syringe pump
Graseby MS 16a syringe driver

WWGH
Alaris (IVAC) P2000 syringe pump
Critikon syringe pump
Graseby 3100 syringe pump
Graseby 500 volumetric pump
Graseby MS 26 or 16a syringe driver

Inventory number of infusion device (Porter to enter when issuing pump)	

Mattress	
PPH	
Patient's PSPS score	
If PSPS 12–16 use	Nimbus III/Cairwave
WWGH	
If PSPS 12–16 use	Pegasus Cairwave
Inventory number of mattress (Porter to enter when issuing mattress)	

Figure 9.2: Equipment request form; PPH=Prince Phillip Hospital; PSPS=Pressure Sore Prediction Score; WWGH=West Wales General Hospital

Appropriate usage

In the 1997 White Paper *The New NHS: Modern, Dependable*, the Government introduced change that would place great emphasis on improving quality of care, treatment and services to the public (Department of Health (DoH), 1997). A new framework of governance was introduced to ensure that clinical management and educational practice is based on scientific evidence (DoH, 1998). This change is implemented at a macro level by the formation of NICE to produce guidelines and assess new technology. More locally, the Health Commission (formally the Commission for Health Improvement) has been created, to monitor the quality of services in both primary and secondary care. At the micro level, clinical governance has made each local chief executive accountable not only for financial management, but also for the quality of the services they provide. Clinical governance incorporates a number of processes, one of which being clinical risk management.

Ensuring that the patient is nursed on the appropriate mattress helps to meet and improve the patient experience through safe and high-quality care. Initially when the static-led approach was introduced in the author's trust, a reduction in inappropriate usage of equipment was noted. This has been monitored through audit over the past 3 years. Recent results indicated that the reduction has maintained inappropriate use at 1.6%. This has been mirrored in the second hospital, where inappropriate use has been reduced from 26% down to 4.6% in the past year since the introduction of the static-led approach.

This year the management of pressure-reducing equipment was cited as an example of good practice in the Welsh Risk Management Standards annual review, an internal document that was part of the trust report.

Prevalence and incidence

Incidence and prevalence surveys reported in the literature suggest that at any one time between 10–15% of the general hospital population is likely to be at risk of pressure ulcers (Gebhardt, 2003). Large variations in prevalence and incidence have been reported across healthcare settings. Incidence is usually defined as the number of persons developing a pressure ulcer after admission divided by all new admissions during the study period (Bergstrom et al, 1994), whereas prevalence is defined as a cross-sectional count of the number of cases at a specific point in time (Philips, 1997).

In this trust, point-prevalence data was traditionally collected twice a year; however, this was not entirely satisfactory as the:

'...day or month when a survey is carried out can markedly affect the results' (Bridel, 1995).

It was decided that an electronic database dedicated to record the weekly incidence and prevalence of pressure ulcers throughout the trust would be used. This database was named SPIDER (Systematic Prevalence and Incidence Date with Enhanced Recording) and was provided by Pegasus as part of the lease contract. While it is difficult to compare prevalence and incidence data with other hospitals owing to variations in study populations and data-collection methods, the regular collection of data has internal benefits. Instant access to prevalence and incidence figures for any period (*Figure 9.3*) and in any specific area of the trust, directorates or wards enables monitoring and comparisons to be made of this trust's performance. Identification of information such as grade, location and origin of ulcers for each clinical area allows specific problems to be highlighted and can be used to determine educational requirements.

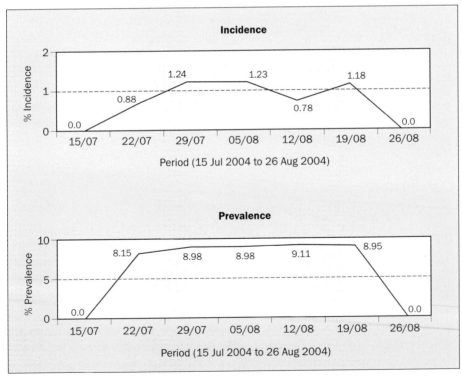

Figure 9.3: Examples of data generated from the electronic database

Figure 9.4 details the anatomical location of pressure ulcers since patient admission to hospital. Timely intervention can be implemented from the identification of early signs of pressure damage.

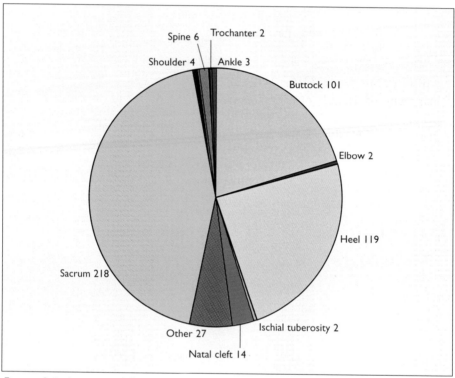

Figure 9.4: Anatomical location of pressure ulcers developing since admission to Carmarthenshire NHS Trust (between 01/01/2003 and 01/01/2004)

Conclusion

The static-led approach was introduced 3 years ago to improve patient care, decrease costs and provide a simple but effective pressure damage prevention programme. It is felt that this objective has been achieved during this time. The system has been regularly monitored since its introduction, and more recently extended to other areas of the trust. Increase in appropriate equipment usage and assessment of patients' risk status as well as a reduction in incidence figures ensures improved clinical effectiveness. At the same time reduced costs allow for a controlled financial budget, which has positive organizational benefits.

References

Bergstrom N, Bennett MA, Carlson CE (1994) *Treatment of Pressure Ulcers. Clinical Practice Guideline No.15.* Department of Health and Human Services, Agency for Health Care Policy and Research, London

Bridel J (1995) Interpreting pressure sore data. *Nurs Stand* **9**(19): 52–4

Collier M (2001) *NT Essential Guide to Wound Assessment.* Emap, London

Collins F (2004) Seating assessment and selection. *J Wound Care/Therapy Weekly Supplement* **13**(5): 9–12

Department of Health (1997) *The New NHS: Modern, Dependable.* The Stationery Office, London

Department of Health (1998) *A First Class Service.* The Stationery Office, London

Gebhardt KS (2003) Cost-effective management of pressure-relieving equipment in a large teaching trust. *J Tissue Viabil* **13**(2): 74–7

Gray DG, Cooper PM, Campbell M (1998) A study of the performance of a pressure-reducing foam mattress after 3 years of use. *J Tissue Viabil* **8**(3): 9–13

Lothian P (1989) Wound care: identifying and protecting patients who may get pressure sores. *Nurs Stand* **4**(4): 26–9

McGough AJ (1999) A systematic review of the effectiveness of risk assessment of pressure sores (unpublished MSc thesis). University of York, York

Maylor ME (2001) Debating the unimportance of pressure-reducing equipment. *Br J Nurs* **10**(15; Tissue Viabil Suppl): S42–S50

National Institute for Clinical Excellence (2001) *Inherited Clinical Guidelines: Pressure Ulcer Risk Assessment and Prevention.* NICE, London

National Institute for Clinical Excellence (2003) *Pressure Ulcer Prevention. Clinical Guideline No.7.* NICE, London

Philips J (1997) *Pressure Sores.* Churchill Livingstone, London: 18

Scott EM (2000) The prevention of pressure ulcers through risk assessment. *J Wound Care* **9**(2): 69–70

Thomas J, James J (2002) Pressure area management: a static-led approach. *Br J Nurs* **11**(14): 967–76

Chapter 10

The benefits of VAC therapy in the management of pressure ulcers

Noleen Smith

This study investigates whether vacuum-assisted closure (VAC) therapy, alginate or hydrocolloid dressings are most effective in the treatment of pressure ulcers. A total of 281 patients were included in this study. The response of each patient's wound was monitored, satisfactory wound closure was examined and the time taken to attain satisfactory wound closure was also taken into consideration. An original analysis of the published data was carried out. Most of the pressure ulcers showed some response in all of the categories investigated, with pressure ulcers in the VAC therapy group showing a greater response in all aspects than those in the other two groups.

Pressure ulcers are described as localized damage to the skin over pressure points, which can extend to underlying muscle and bone (Dealey, 1994). They are most prominent over areas such as the sacrum, heels, hips and elbows (Lewis, 1997). Susceptibility to pressure ulcers increases in patients who are immobile for long periods, such as older people, patients with severe, acute illnesses and patients with neurological problems, e.g. spinal cord injuries (Jacquot et al, 1999).

Pressure ulcers are prevalent in hospital situations, nursing homes and in patients' own homes. The number of patients suffering with chronic, non-healing wounds such as pressure ulcers is rising, and they are more common in people over 60 years of age (Goodridge et al, 1998). This increasing prevalence puts great strain on all NHS resources. The cost of treating pressure ulcers has a range of £60 million–£200 million per year (Ivory, 1999). The cost of preventing them is thought to have the same range. This leads to a range of £120 million–£400 million per year for the care of pressure ulcers (Clay, 2000).

Optimum wound healing depends on many factors including the most effective dressing, not only in terms of the wound closure achieved but also the ability of the dressing to achieve satisfactory wound closure in the shortest time-frame (Lewis, 1998). The objectives of any treatment are to obtain satisfactory wound closure in the shortest time before direct closure or surgery can achieve total wound closure (Dealey, 1994).

Direct closure is useful if the wound is small; however, if the wound is exceptionally large, sometimes the only way to close the wound is to use a fasciocutaneous or myocutaneous flap (Mathes and Nahai, 1982). A fasciocutaneous flap makes use of the epidermis, dermis and fascia, as well as incorporating blood vessels to keep the flap alive. This flap is then rotated from its original position to the area that it needs to cover. A myocutaneous flap is used for deeper wounds or areas that require more padding. A myocutaneous flap makes use of the epidermis, dermis and fascia, as well as the muscle and blood vessels.

Surgery should be the last resort and is usually only used on very large wounds or wounds that refuse to heal (Mathes and Nahai, 1982).

Treatment of pressure ulcers

VAC therapy

Pressure ulcers have been managed in various ways over the years. The development of vacuum-assisted closure (VAC) therapy is one of the most recent developments in the treatment of chronic wounds (Miller and Glover, 1999). VAC therapy facilitates wound management in many circumstances. It is recommended in deep chronic wounds with moderate to high exudate levels. These include pressure ulcers, abscesses and deep wounds owing to trauma (Argenta and Morykwas, 1997).

VAC therapy uses the application of topical negative pressure (TNP) across the wound surface and includes the use of a foam dressing (Miller and Glover, 1999). The foam dressing needs to be of the open-pore variety, cut to shape and inserted into the wound so that direct contact with the wound surface is attained. A transparent adhesive dressing is placed over the foam in order to create a controlled, closed wound environment. TNP is then applied using a vacuum pump across the wound via a drainage tube placed within the foam. This drainage tube must not rest on a bony surface as it will facilitate pressure ulcer formation (Miller and Glover, 1999).

VAC therapy creates a hypoxic environment within the wound bed, ensuring that aerobic bacteria cannot survive. TNP applied across the wound forces the microcirculation to regenerate quickly and encourages capillary growth (angiogenesis). As TNP draws blood into the wound bed, it brings with it growth factors and macrophages to an area depleted in bacterial contamination. It also increases oxygen availability needed for tissue regeneration. TNP removes slough and loose necrotic material from the wound, cleaning the wound and ensuring a good blood supply. A clean wound and good blood supply encourages the formation of granulation tissue (encouraging wound closure) and ensures that white blood cells are supplied with necessary oxygen via the bloodstream, while ensuring that anaerobic bacteria in the wound bed die (Miller and Glover, 1999).

VAC therapy has been shown to reduce the colonization of bacteria (Miller and Glover, 1999). It provides a moist wound environment, which is essential for wound healing as poorly perfused, traumatized tissue that is allowed to dehydrate will transform from an area of 'stasis' to one of 'necrosis', leading to further tissue loss and unpleasant scar formation (Banwell, 1999). A wet environment also increases healing rates and reduces inflammation (Svensjö et al, 2000). The main aim of VAC therapy is to achieve an increase in patient comfort while decreasing patient morbidity (Argenta and Morykwas, 1997).

Hydrocolloid dressings

Hydrocolloid dressings contain gel-forming agents, such as sodium carboxymethylcellulose and gelatin. This gel is combined with elastomers and adhesives and applied to a foam or film, forming the complete dressing. Hydrocolloid dressings work as follows: the dressing is applied to the wound, comes into contact with the exudate and interacts with the exudate to form a gel (Williams, 1996). The gel forms a moist environment on the surface of the wound. Hydrocolloid dressings do not cause maceration of the surrounding skin and actually promote the formation of granulation tissue (Williams, 1996). These dressings are designed to deal with mild to moderately exuding wounds.

Alginate dressings

Alginate dressings (extracted from seaweed) function by interacting with wound exudate to form a hydrophilic gel, thus providing a moist wound environment (Thomas et al, 1997). They reduce blood loss and healing times significantly (Thomas, 2000). Haemostatic activity is caused by platelet activation and whole-blood coagulation initiated by the exchange of calcium ions for sodium ions in the blood (Thomas et al, 1997). This calcium acts as factor IV in haemostasis. Alginate dressings vary in weight and can absorb 15–20 times their own weight of exudate. A plain sheet of alginate is placed on the wound surface then covered with a suitable secondary dressing. The fact that alginate dressings absorb exudate, reduce bacterial colonization and encourage healing by promoting the formation of granulation tissue makes them suitable for treating pressure ulcers (Thomas et al, 1997). Alginate dressings can also be used to cover split skin grafts (Hormbrey et al, 2003).

Aim

The aim of this study was to determine which of the treatments discussed above most benefit the patient with pressure ulcers in terms of overall outcome, by examining the results of previously published studies into their efficacy.

Method

This study made use of published data in order to investigate VAC therapy, hydrocolloid dressings and alginate dressings with the aim of reaching a conclusion as to which of these are most effective in the treatment of pressure ulcers. The three determining factors were:

■ Whether the wound responds to the dressing, i.e. is there any sign of healing such as the presence of granulation tissue?
■ Whether the wound attains satisfactory closure requiring little or no further treatment
■ Which dressing obtains satisfactory results in the shortest time-frame (observations took place over approximately 16 weeks).

Extensive research was undertaken to obtain a select few journal articles that met the criteria for this study. The following databases were searched: BIOSIS, Medline, Cochrane Library and OVID. The published articles obtained had to eliminate as much bias as possible, and they had to be similar in terms of the factors listed in *Table 10.1*.

Table 10.1: Comparison criteria for the studies chosen

- The factors considered, i.e. response of the wound to the dressing used (were there any signs of healing or were there no signs of healing?); satisfactory closure of the wound (satisfactory wound closure was deemed to be when little or no further treatment was needed) and the time-frame needed to attain satisfactory closure (range of <3 weeks–≥16 weeks)

- Patient numbers — greater than 40 in all studies

- Pressure ulcer grading — all those studied had approximately the same grading: grade 2–4 (Moody et al, 1993)

Three journal articles were selected. These are referenced in full below for the benefit of the reader:

- Thomas S, Banks V, Bale S et al (1997) A comparison of two dressings in the management of chronic wounds. *J Wound Care* **6**: 383–6
- Sayag J, Meaume S, Bohbot S (1996) Healing properties of calcium alginate dressings. *J Wound Care* **5**: 357–62
- Argenta LC, Morykwas MJ (1997) Vacuum-assisted closure: a new method for wound control and treatment: clinical experience. *Ann Plast Surg* **38**: 563–76.

Data was gathered from these articles and grouped together as follows:

- Response or lack of response towards treatment
- Satisfactory wound closure
- Time-frame required to achieve satisfactory wound closure.

When working with the data for response/lack of response, a χ^2 test was used. The χ^2 test was carried out between the three groups and again between each of the groups in pairs (i.e. VAC and hydrocolloid, VAC and alginate and hydrocolloid and alginate). With regard to the data for the time period required to achieve satisfactory wound closure, a Kruskal–Wallis non-parametric analysis of variance (ANOVA) test was used. It must be noted that a Kruskal–Wallis ANOVA test was not only carried out on the three groups together, but also was done on two groups at a time in order to determine if there was any statistically significant difference between them. The statistical tests were carried out using the computer software package Statistical Package for the Social Sciences (SPSS).

Results

When pressure ulcers were treated with VAC therapy, most of the pressure ulcers attained satisfactory wound closure. Pressure ulcers treated with a hydrocolloid dressing had satisfactory results, with approximately 33% (16/48)

Table 10.2: Comparison of wound response and satisfactory wound closure between the three treatment types				
	Number of wounds responding	%	Number of wounds attaining satisfactory closure	%
VAC therapy	137/141	97	131/141	93
Alginate dressing	68/92	74	0/92	0
Hydrocolloid dressing	16/48	33	30/48	63

of the pressure ulcers in this group attaining satisfactory wound closure. Pressure ulcers that were treated with alginate dressings showed that 0% reached a satisfactory wound closure (*Table 10.2*).

VAC therapy was able to heal wounds in a shorter period of time than the other two treatments, but the alginate dressings were better in this respect than the hydrocolloid dressing. Even though none of the alginate-treated wounds attained satisfactory closure (deemed to be closure of 60–80%, i.e. suitable for primary closure or a little further treatment), many of the hydrocolloid-treated wounds were at the same stage of closure or worse than the alginate dressing, although some did attain satisfactory closure. Most pressure ulcers in all three groups attained a satisfactory percentage closure within 10 weeks (*Table 10.3*).

Most of the pressure ulcers treated with the VAC therapy attained satisfactory results in the shortest time (3–4 weeks). Of the pressure ulcers treated with alginate dressings, 37% showed good signs of healing although they did not reach satisfactory wound closure where little or no further

Table 10.3: Comparison of the treatment with regard to the time taken to achieve satisfactory signs of wound healing

Time taken to attain satisfactory closure (weeks)	VAC therapy	Alginate dressing	Hydrocolloid dressing
<3 weeks	43	0	0
3–4 weeks	55	34	0
5–10 weeks	27	38	38
10–15 weeks	10	0	0
≥16 weeks	6	20	10
Total	*141*	*92*	*48*

treatment was needed. This does not mean that they were far off from this stage; these wounds may have just missed the mark in the time-frame. Pressure ulcers treated with alginate dressings showed satisfactory signs of healing within 3–4 weeks. No pressure ulcers healed in 3–4 weeks in the hydrocolloid dressing group; they all seemed to pick up after this and to show signs of healing. Alginate dressings were shown to elicit a faster healing response than hydrocolloid dressings, but a slower healing response than VAC therapy.

Table 10.4 explains statistically that there is a difference in efficacy between the three dressing types with regard to wound response. There is also

Table 10.4: Statistical results when comparing the three treatment types in all three categories

Category	VAC, alginate, hydrocolloid	VAC and alginate	VAC and hydrocolloid	Alginate and hydrocolloid
Wound response	$P \leq 0.025$	$P > 0.05$	$P \leq 0.001$	$P > 0.05$
Satisfactory wound closure	$P \leq 0.000$	$P \leq 0.000$	$P \leq 0.002$	$P \leq 0.000$
Time taken to attain satisfactory wound closure	$P \leq 0.000$	$P \leq 0.000$	$P \leq 0.000$	$P \leq 0.039$

a statistically significant difference between VAC therapy and hydrocolloid dressings. There is no statistically significant difference between the VAC therapy and alginate dressings or the alginate and hydrocolloid dressings with regard to wound response.

Table 10.4 also shows that there is a statistically significant difference between the three dressings when compared against one another and in the pair analysis in terms of satisfactory wound closure. The same thing is seen with regard to the time taken to attain satisfactory signs of healing.

Discussion

The treatment that was most successful in all of the areas examined, i.e. response of the wound, satisfactory wound closure and time taken to achieve satisfactory wound closure, was VAC therapy. These observations indicate that for pressure ulcers of grades 2–4, VAC therapy aids wound healing to a greater extent than alginate or hydrocolloid dressings. It is not known exactly how it accomplishes these results. It is postulated that no single mechanism of VAC therapy is responsible for its success, but it is rather a combination of all the mechanisms (Banwell, 1999). Some advantages of VAC therapy include:

■ Removing exudate
■ Increasing blood supply to the wound
■ Reducing oedema of the wound
■ Exerting mechanical stress on the wound surface and edges
■ Decreasing bacterial colonization rates
■ Providing occlusion to the wound (Banwell, 1999).

VAC therapy has also been found to reduce the pain experienced by the patient and reduce the cost of treatment (Banwell, 1999). Patients being treated with VAC therapy can be treated as outpatients, thereby reducing hospitalization costs (Banwell, 1999). VAC therapy also reduces the need for further extensive treatments such as major surgery, by healing some pressure ulcers to an extent where primary closure or a split-skin graft may be all that is needed (Argenta and Morykwas, 1997).

Successful wound healing relies on certain criteria. One of these is a good blood supply to the wound while it is healing (Reed, 1998). Vascular changes early on in the wound-healing process encourage the presence of macrophages and neutrophils (Solomon et al, 1990). Macrophages (a type of leucocyte) are specialized cells that engulf large particles, such as bacteria, yeast and dying cells, by phagocytosis. Neutrophils make up 55–70% of all the leucocytes and are attracted to sites of injury and infection, where they adhere to vessel walls in a process known as margination. They then migrate into the surrounding tissue and engulf bacteria by phagocytosis (Solomon et al, 1990).

TNP increases local blood flow and decreases oedema; therefore, hypoxic conditions are minimized, i.e. the wound is satisfactorily oxygenated, creating a favourable wound environment (Banwell, 1999). Using Doppler flowmetry, it is shown that at pressures of less than 150 mmHg, dermal blood flow is increased by up to four times when using VAC therapy (Banwell, 1999). These pressures work by creating a gradient via a direct mechanical effect, i.e. pulling blood through the vessels. This active gradient increases the blood supply to the wound. Tissue oedema impedes the vascular supply of the wound and if the vascular supply is already tenuous the presence of oedema causes further complications. TNP plays an active role in removing/decreasing tissue oedema by actively removing the interstitial fluid and, therefore, aids blood flow to the wound (Banwell, 1999).

TNP exerts mechanical stress on the wound surface and edges. This mechanical stress has a direct effect on cellular activity (mitosis is encouraged), especially angiogenesis (Banwell, 1999). Angiogenesis increases blood flow to the wound and, in so doing, aids the wound-healing process as previously discussed. TNP therefore aids wound closure by mechanical stress. Using the foam suction dressing, a centripetal force (directed to the centre of the wound) is created that draws the edges of the wound together. The stretching of skin beyond its inherent elasticity is known as mechanical creep. VAC therapy initiates mechanical creep and so encourages wound healing (Banwell, 1999).

Both alginate dressings and VAC therapy remove exudate. However, VAC therapy does not become saturated. The amount of exudate that the alginate dressing is holding will, at some point, exceed the 'holding' capacity of the dressing and the dressing will no longer be able to absorb exudate (Heenan, 1998). As the wound exudate is being completely removed into a separate container in the case of VAC therapy, the 'holding' capacity of VAC therapy is higher than that of the alginate dressing (Williams, 1998).

Hydrocolloid dressings do remove a certain amount of wound exudate. The hydrocolloid dressing reacts with the wound exudate in order to form a gel, which produces a favourable moist wound environment. Owing to the formation of this hydrophilic gel, excess wound exudate is removed and this aids wound healing (Williams, 1996). However, hydrocolloid dressings are only suitable for use in the treatment of light to moderately exuding wounds, as they become overwhelmed by exudate after a couple of days when applied to wounds that produce a large amount of exudate (Banks et al, 1994).

Alginate dressings do not exert any pressure on the wound; therefore, they do not increase the local blood flow, which is one of the factors that is thought to aid in the healing of the wound. However, they do affect the vascularity of the wound (Iwai, 1996) and provide a barrier against contamination. Once the alginate dressing is in place, bacterial colonization rates are stable as alginate dressings are impermeable to bacteria. Although bacteria remain in the wound and antibiotics are required to control the rate of colonization, the spread of bacterial infection is prevented (Sayag et al, 1996). Alginate dressings decrease blood loss within the wound. It has been shown that haemostatic activity is caused by platelet activation and whole blood coagulation, which is initiated by the exchange of calcium ions for sodium ions within the blood owing to the fact that some alginate dressings contain calcium ions, i.e. calcium alginate dressings. This means that clotting is encouraged and blood loss is decreased, which aids in the healing of the wound (Thomas, 1992).

Hydrocolloid dressings do not exert pressure on the wound; therefore, they have no effect on the vascularity of the wound (Williams, 1996). The lack of pressure and therefore the lack of influence on local blood flow means that these dressings are unable to increase oxygenation of the wound or to encourage the presence of macrophages and neutrophils to combat infection (Banks et al, 1994). Hydrocolloid dressings do not affect the vascularity of the wound; alginate dressings do, however, and therefore have an additional wound-healing property. Satisfactory wound closure is different to attaining satisfactory percentage closure. The percentage closure, e.g. 60–80%, is considered to show satisfactory wound healing. So although no alginate-treated wounds attained satisfactory closure they did show signs of satisfactory healing and may have healed completely, but not in the time-frame of this study.

According to Banwell (1999), VAC therapy decreases bacterial colonization rates in wounds. This decrease is claimed to be caused by an increased blood flow, which oxygenates the area, and an increase in the presence of macrophages and neutrophils, which rid the wound of bacteria via phagocytosis. The removal of slough and exudate decreases the ability of bacteria to colonize the wound. What is unknown is whether the overall effect is a result of direct removal of bacteria via suction or an increase in the local vascular supply and therefore an increase in the oxygen content and leucocyte availability.

Chronic wound exudate contains high levels of proteolytic enzymes that suppress the formation of keratinocytes, endothelial cells and fibroblasts, thus inhibiting wound healing. VAC therapy removes wound exudate, and in so doing helps to promote healing of the wound (Banwell, 1999). An additional benefit of this therapy is through the application of a semi-permeable film, e.g.

Opsite. This film helps retain the foam dressing in the wound, provides an airtight seal (avoiding loss of vacuum) (Banwell, 1999) and facilitates moist wound healing, thus increasing the rate of epidermal resurfacing and formation of granulation tissue.

Other beneficial effects of occlusion include: prevention of wound desiccation, prevention of cell death, accelerated angiogenesis, increased breakdown of dead tissues and fibrin, and an increase in the chance of growth factors interacting with their target cells. Pain is also reduced when occlusion takes place (Banwell, 1999).

Hydrocolloid dressings do not decrease tissue oedema whether in the active or the passive role. If a hydrocolloid dressing is applied to a vascularly compromised wound, the dressing will not aid in correcting or alleviating the situation. The blood supply will continue to be tenuous if the hydrocolloid dressing is left *in situ* (Bale et al, 1997). With regard to decreasing tissue oedema, the hydrocolloid dressing and alginate dressing are on a par with one another in that they exert no effect in this respect.

Hydrocolloid dressings maintain a stable bacterial population. Once a species is present in a wound it remains, although numbers do not escalate exceedingly. *Pseudomonas spp.*, however, has been shown to be inhibited by the presence of the hydrocolloid dressing (Heenan, 1998). Once again, antibiotics are required to prevent bacterial colonization. The hydrocolloid dressing is on a par with the alginate dressing in this respect. Bacteria can affect the healing rate of the wound by increasing tissue death and therefore increasing tissue loss (Heenan, 1998).

Hydrocolloid dressings do remove a certain amount of wound exudate (Williams, 1996). They are suitable for use in the treatment of light to moderately exuding wounds as they become overwhelmed by exudate when applied to wounds that produce a large amount (Banks et al, 1994). This means that some of the exudate will remain in the wound and will inhibit wound healing because of the presence of excess proteolytic enzymes (Kim et al, 1996). Therefore, the alginate and VAC therapy surpass the ability of the hydrocolloid dressing in respect to the removal of large amounts of exudate. This study included wounds that were moderate to high in the amount of exudate they produced. Therefore, the VAC therapy and the alginate dressings should exhibit better healing results than the hydrocolloid dressing, as they are able to handle large volumes of exudate.

Hydrocolloid dressings can be occluded; this occlusion aids in maintaining a moist wound environment and encourages the formation of granulation tissue (Ichioka et al, 1998).

Hydrocolloid and alginate dressings exert a small amount of mechanical stress on the edges of the wound by having an adhesive edge that may pull slightly at the wound edges and, therefore, encourage mitosis. However, the mechanical forces exerted by the hydrocolloid and alginate dressings are minimal when compared with the forces exerted by VAC therapy.

Limitations of study

Analyzing the results of three separate studies carried out by different people in different ways will cause bias, but the studies were chosen in order to limit as much bias as possible. In this study there are bound to be experimental errors, for example both the VAC therapy and the alginate dressing are best suited for moderate to high exudating wounds, whereas the hydrocolloid dressing is best suited for wounds that have a relatively low volume of exudate (Banks et al, 1994). The wounds included in this study were of the moderate to high exudate-producing wounds, and therefore it is relatively unfair to include the hydrocolloid dressing when it is known that it cannot cope with the amount of exudate experienced in this study. This may be why the hydrocolloid dressing results were poor compared with the other two. However, in some aspects the hydrocolloid dressing did fare better than the alginate dressing. VAC therapy appeared more effective than the alginate and hydrocolloid dressings, even when the pressure ulcers included were of a higher grade. This may be an unfair assumption because of the fact that the study included less active dressings, i.e. hydrocolloid and alginate dressings with the extremely active VAC therapy.

It cannot be assumed that VAC therapy should be used on all pressure ulcers, and it is the nurse's decision to determine the dressing of choice based on the severity and the position of the wound. It must also be noted that VAC therapy is not a replacement for surgery, but merely decreases the extent of the surgery if needed in the future. For extremely large pressure ulcers, extensive surgery may be required in the form of fasciocutaneous or musculocutaneous flaps in order to cover large, open wounds that may have exposed vessels or bony protuberances.

Another factor that may add bias is the health of the patient being treated. Underlying health problems were not disclosed in the three studies and therefore are not in this study. This could result in bias and, therefore, effect the overall outcome of the study.

Conclusion

It has been shown that VAC therapy surpasses both the alginate and hydrocolloid dressings in terms of response of wounds to treatment, satisfactory closure and the time taken to achieve these results. Although the alginate dressing did not achieve satisfactory wound closure, it did initiate wound response and wounds did heal but not to the extent that primary closure or no further treatment was needed (within the time-frame of this study). Hydrocolloid dressings did achieve some satisfactory wound closure, but on the whole most of the wounds treated with this dressing lay in the same range as those treated with alginate dressings. Alginate dressings have better wound-healing capabilities than the hydrocolloid dressing and are able to handle moderate to severely exuding wounds better than hydrocolloid dressings. This indicates that for moderate to severely exuding wounds, VAC therapy and alginate dressings are a better choice than hydrocolloid dressings, and VAC therapy is a better choice than the alginate dressing.

References

Argenta LC, Morykwas MJ (1997) Vacuum-assisted closure: a new method for wound control and treatment: clinical experience. *Ann Plast Surg* **38**(6): 563–76

Bale S, Squires D, Varnon T, Walker A, Benbow M, Harding KG (1997) A comparison of two dressings in pressure sore management. *J Wound Care* **6:** 463–6

Banks V, Bale S, Harding K (1994) The use of two dressings for moderately exuding pressure sores. *J Wound Care* **3:** 132–4

Banwell PE (1999) Topical negative pressure therapy in wound care. *J Wound Care* **8:** 79–84

Clay M (2000) Pressure sore prevention in nursing homes. *Nurs Stand* **14**(44): 45–50

Dealey C (1994) *The Care of Wounds.* Blackwell Science, London

Goodridge DM, Sloan JA, LeDoyen YM, McKenzie JA, Knight WE, Gayari M (1998) Risk-assessment scores, prevention strategies and the incidence of pressure ulcers among the elderly in four Canadian health-care facilities. *Can J Nurs Res* **30**(2): 23–44

Heenan A (1998) *Frequently Asked Questions: Hydrocolloid Dressings.* Word Wide Wounds (www.worldwidewounds.com/1998/april/Hydrocolloid-FAQ/hydrocolloid-questions.html) (last accessed 25 November 2004)

Hormbrey E, Pandya A, Giele H (2003) Adhesive retention dressings are more comfortable than alginate dressings on split-skin-graft donor sites. *Br J Plast Surg* **56**(5): 498–503

Ichioka S, Harii K, Nakahara M, Sato Y (1998) An experimental comparison of hydrocolloid and alginate dressings and the effect of calcium ions in the behaviour of alginate gel. *Scand J Plast Reconstr Surg Hand Surg* **32**(3): 311–16

Ivory P (1999) The lurking dangers of pressure sores. *Quest* **6**(1): 1–6

Iwai T (1996) Critical limb ischaemia. *Nippon Geka Gakka Zasshi* (*Journal of Japanese Surgical Society*) **97**(7): 486–91

Jacquot JM, Pelissier J, Finels H, Strubel D (1999) Epidemiology and cost of pressure sores in the aged. *Presse Med* **28**: 1854–60

Kim YC, Shin JC, Park CI, Oh SH, Choi SM, Kim YS (1996) Efficacy of hydrocolloid occlusive dressing technique in decubitus ulcer treatment: a comparative study. *Yonsei Med J* **37**(3): 181–5

Lewis BK (1997) Nutrition and age in the aetiology of pressure sores. *J Wound Care* **6:** 41–2

Lewis BK (1998) Nutrient intake and the risk of pressure sore development in older patients. *J Wound Care* **7:** 31–5

Mathes SJ, Nahai F (1982) *Clinical Applications for Muscle and Myocutaneous Flaps.* CV Mosby, St Louis, Missouri

Miller M, Glover D (1999) *Wound Management: Theory and Practice.* The Friary Press, London

Moody M, Clark J, Barbenel J et al (1993) *Pressure Sores: A Key Quality Indicator.* Department of Health, London

Reed MJ (1998) Wound repair in older patients: preventing problems and managing the healing. *Geriatrics* **53**(5): 88–94

Sayag J, Meaume S, Bohbot S (1996) Healing properties of calcium alginate dressings. *J Wound Care* **5:** 357–62

Solomon EP, Schmidt RR, Adragna PJ (1990) *Human Anatomy and Physiology.* 2nd edn. Saunders College Publications, Fort Worth

Svensjö T, Pomahac B, Yao F, Slama J, Eriksson E (2000) Accelerated healing of full-thickness wounds in a wet environment. *Plast Reconstr Surg* **106:** 602–12

Thomas S (1992) Alginates: a guide to the properties and uses of the different alginate dressings available today. *J Wound Care* **1**(1): 29–32

Thomas S (2000) Alginate dressings in surgery and wound management — part 1. *J Wound Care* **9**(2): 56–60

Thomas S, Banks V, Bale S et al (1997) A comparison of two dressings in the management of chronic wounds. *J Wound Care* **6:** 383–6

Williams C (1996) Tegasorb hydrocolloid dressing: advanced formulation. *Br J Nurs* **5:** 1271–2

Williams C (1998) Melgisorb: a highly absorbent calcium/sodium alginate dressing. *Br J Nurs* **7:** 975–6

Chapter 11

TIME principles of chronic wound bed preparation and treatment

Caroline Dowsett, Elizabeth Ayello

Managing chronic wounds has progressed from merely assessing the wound to understanding the underlying cellular abnormalities and associated clinical problems. The concept of wound bed preparation offers a systematic approach to removing barriers to healing, such as tissue (non-viable), infection/inflammation, moisture (imbalance) and edge (non-advancing or undermining). The principles of wound bed preparation as outlined in the tissue, infection, moisure, edge (TIME) table are explained in this chapter, with examples and recommended treatment interventions. The TIME table is recommended for use at the bedside when assessing patients with wounds.

Wound bed preparation is a relatively new concept in wound care, although the elements that make up the concept are not. This chapter provides an overview of the concept as it relates to practice, and introduces the principles of TIME:

- Tissue
- Infection
- Moisture
- Edge.

Wound bed preparation is the management of a wound to accelerate endogenous healing or to facilitate the effectiveness of other therapeutic measures (Falanga, 2000; Schultz et al, 2003). Wound bed preparation allows healthcare professionals to define the steps involved in the management of chronic wounds through an understanding of the basic science underlying the problems. It is an approach that should be considered for all wounds that are not progressing to normal healing (Schultz et al, 2003).

Wound healing is a complex series of events that are interlinked and dependent on one another and can be defined as the physiological processes by which the body replaces and restores function to damaged tissue (Tortora and Grabowski, 2000). Acute wounds usually follow a well-defined process described as: coagulation; inflammation; cell proliferation and repair of the matrix; and epithelialization and remodelling of scar tissue (Schultz et al, 2003). These stages overlap and the entire wound-healing process can take several months.

In the past, the acute wound-healing model has been applied to chronic wounds, but it is now known that chronic wound healing is different from acute wound healing. Chronic wounds become 'stuck' in the inflammatory and proliferative phases of healing (Ennis and Meneses, 2000), which delays healing. The epidermis fails to migrate across the wound tissue and there is hyperproliferation at the wound margins, which interferes with normal cellular migration over the wound bed (Schultz et al, 2003).

In chronic wounds there appears to be an overproduction of matrix molecules resulting from underlying cellular dysfunction and disregulation (Falanga et al, 1994). Fibrinogen and fibrin are also common in chronic wounds, and it is thought that these and other macromolecules scavenge growth factors and other molecules involved in promoting wound repair (Falanga, 2000). So, while there may be a large number of growth factors within the wound, these can become trapped and therefore unavailable to the wound-repair process.

Chronic wound fluid is also biochemically distinct from acute wound fluid; it slows down, or even blocks the proliferation of cells, such as keratinocytes, fibroblasts and endothelial cells, which are essential for the wound-healing process (Schultz et al, 2003).

The principles of wound bed preparation

In a wound that fails to heal there is often a complex mix of local and host factors that need to be assessed and treated. A full and detailed patient assessment will highlight the underlying aetiology of the wound and other factors that may impede healing, such as poor nutrition and pain (Dealey, 2002). The underlying cause will need to be addressed if wound bed preparation is to be successful. Wound bed preparation is a way of focusing systematically on all of the critical components of a non-healing wound to identify the possible cause of the problem. It is a concept that links treatment

Table 11.1: The TIME principles of wound bed preparation (WBP)

CLINICAL OBSERVATIONS	PROPOSED PATHOPHYSIOLOGY	WBP CLINICAL ACTIONS	EFFECT OF WBP ACTIONS	CLINICAL OUTCOME
TISSUE NON-VIABLE OR DEFICIENT	Defective matrix and cell debris impair healing	Debridement (episodic or continuous) • autolytic, sharp surgical, enzymatic, mechanical • biological agents	Restoration of wound base and functional extracellular matrix proteins	Viable wound base
INFECTION OR INFLAMMATION	High bacterial counts or prolonged inflammation ↑ inflammatory cytokines ↑ protease activity ↓ growth factor activity	Remove infected foci Topical/systemic • antimicrobials • anti-inflammatories • protease inhibition	Low bacterial counts or controlled inflammation: ↓ inflammatory cytokines ↓ protease activity ↑ growth factor activity	Bacterial balance and reduced inflammation
MOISTURE IMBALANCE	Desiccation slows epithelial cell migration Excessive fluid causes maceration of wound margin	Apply moisture-balancing dressings Compression, negative pressure or other methods of removing fluid	Restored epithelial cell migration, desiccation avoided Oedema, excessive fluid controlled, maceration avoided	Moisture balance
EDGE OF WOUND – NON ADVANCING OR UNDERMINED	Non-migrating keratinocytes Non-responsive wound cells and abnormalities in extracellular matrix or abnormal protease activity	Reassess cause or consider corrective therapies • debridement • skin grafts • biological agents • adjunctive therapies	Migrating keratinocytes and responsive wound cells. Restoration of appropriate protease profile	Advancing edge of wound

From Schultz et al (2003)

to the cause of the wound by focusing on the components of local wound care (Sibbald et al, 2000): debridement, bacterial balance and moisture balance.

The TIME table (*Table 11.1*) illustrates in a simple way the link between clinical observations and underlying cellular abnormalities, and the effects of clinical interventions at a cellular level.

A useful way of remembering the process of wound bed preparation is to use the acronym shown in this table, based on the observable characteristics of non-healing wounds (Schultz et al, 2003):

- T — for tissue that is non-viable or deficient
- I — for infection/inflammation
- M — for moisture imbalance, which must be corrected
- E — for edge, which is not advancing across the wound bed.

Table 11.1 has been designed to help the wound care practitioner make a systematic interpretation of the observable characteristics of a wound and to decide on the most appropriate intervention. The first column lists the clinical signs of a non-healing wound. As growth factors, senescent cells or fibroblasts cannot be seen with the naked eye, the clinician needs clear, visible signs that can be assessed at the bedside. The second column highlights the proposed pathophysiology of that clinical observation. Column three and four suggest the clinical actions that need to be taken and the effects of these actions. The final column is for clinical outcomes, which are objective and measurable.

Wound bed preparation together with TIME have led to an increased awareness of the need for systematic approaches to wound management. One concept that complements wound bed preparation and TIME is that of Applied Wound Management (Gray et al, 2005), which proposes a systematic approach at a practical level by using three continuums — healing, infection and exudate. The advantage of this complementary approach is that it not only supports clinical decision-making, but can also facilitate clinical audit.

T for tissue: dealing with non-viable tissue

Non-viable tissue, such as slough or necrosis, delays wound healing and is a focus for infection. The clinician needs to assess the wound and intervene using the TIME table:

- Clinical sign or symptom — non-viable, deficient tissue
- Underlying problem — impedes actions of growth factors, blocks cellular migration, provides a focus for continued infection and inflammation
- Intervention — debridement, repeated if necessary.

There are two important factors in considering tissue as a key element of wound bed preparation:

- To promote the growth of healthy tissue
- To clear away necrotic or non-viable tissue from the wound bed.

For the promotion of healthy tissue growth, a well-vascularized wound bed is essential (Schultz et al, 2003). Often this means both treatment of the wound bed and a consideration of the overall factors that have compromised the blood supply to the wound. It is also essential to clear away the non-viable tissue that is preventing good tissue growth (Steed et al, 1996).

Devitalized, necrotic tissue (*Figure 11.1*) provides a focus for infection, prolongs the inflammatory phase, mechanically obstructs contraction and impedes re-epithelialization (Baharestani, 1999).

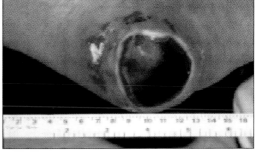

Figure 11.1: A necrotic wound

It may also mask underlying fluid collections or abscesses and make it difficult to evaluate wound depth. If the wound clearly contains non-viable or deficient tissue, a method of removing it should be considered in order to promote healing and reduce the risk of local infection (Vowden and Vowden, 1999; Fairbairn et al, 2002). This process is usually referred to as debridement, which is widely used to leave a clean surface that will heal relatively easily.

Chronic wounds are likely to require ongoing maintenance debridement rather than a single intervention (Falanga, 2002). The underlying pathogenic abnormalities in chronic wounds cause a continual build-up of necrotic tissue, and regular debridement may be necessary to reduce the necrotic burden and achieve healthy granulation tissue. Debridement also reduces wound contamination and therefore reduces tissue destruction (Sibbald et al, 2000).

In the early stages of wound healing, debridement occurs autolytically through the action of enzymes (including elastase, collagenase, myeloperoxidase, acid hydrolase and lysosomes). At the same time, inhibitors are released by wound cells to restrict the debridement action to the wound bed, minimizing damage to intact tissue at the wound edge (Schultz et al, 2003). Debridement using surgical, enzymatic, autolytic or mechanical methods is often all that is required to promote the first step in the healing process. Although debridement occurs naturally, assisted debridement accelerates the wound-healing process (Sibbald et al, 2000).

Five methods of debridement are available, each with their own advantages and limitations (O'Brien, 2002). The methods that are most efficient at the removal of debris may, at the same time, be the most detrimental to fragile new growth, and more than one method may be appropriate.

The five methods are:

- Autolytic
- Surgical/sharp
- Enzymatic
- Mechanical
- Biological.

The chosen method of debridement will depend on the patient characteristics and preferences, the knowledge and skills of the clinician and the resources available. *Table 11.2* highlights the clinical considerations. The method/methods of debridement used should be evidence-based and evaluated in terms of their effectiveness. Specialist advice should be sought from the tissue viability specialist or wound care specialist where the wound is failing to debride with the chosen method, or when the clinician lacks the knowledge and skills to carry out the chosen method of debridement.

Table 11.2: Clinical considerations when choosing a method of debridement

Wound

Aetiology; location; extent of tissue damage; type of tissue involvement; size and extent of devitalized tissue; amount of exudate production

Practical considerations

Clinical expertise and professional accountability; availability of resources; time available; cost-effectiveness; patients' wishes

From Flanagan (1997)

I or infection: resolution of bacterial imbalance

Infection in a wound causes pain and discomfort for the patient — delayed wound healing can be life-threatening. The clinician needs to assess for clinical signs and symptoms of infection and intervene using the TIME table:

Table 11.3: Signs and symptoms of superficial and deep tissue infection

Superficial	Non-healing; friable granulation tissue that bleeds easily; exuberant bright red granulation; increased exudate or discharge; new areas of necrosis in base; breakdown of granulation tissue; odour
Deep	Pain (other than usually reported); increased size; warmth (abnormal/elevated temperature); erythema >1–2 cm; probes to bone or bone exposed

From Sibbald et al (2000)

- Clinical sign or symptom (outlined in *Table 11.3*)
- Underlying problem — infection caused by high levels of bacteria
- Intervention — debridement, antimicrobials, anti-inflammatories.

All chronic wounds contain bacteria, and their presence in a wound does not necessarily indicate that infection has occurred or that wound healing will be impaired (Kerstein, 1997; Dow et al, 1999). However, where infection is present in a wound, as shown in *Figure 11.2*, it delays wound healing through the maintenance of a proinflammatory environment (Schultz et al, 2003). The signs and symptoms of superficial and deep tissue infection are outlined in *Table 11.3* above.

When a wound is infected it contains replicating micro-organisms that cause injury to the host. In an acute wound, infection is met by a rapid inflammatory response that is initiated by the release of cytokines and growth

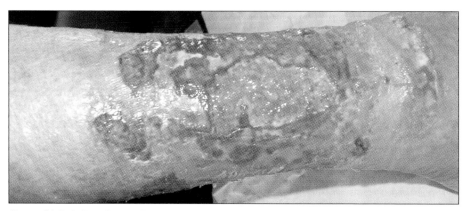

Figure 11.2: Infected wound

factors (Dow et al, 1999). The inflammatory cascade produces vasodilation and a significant increase of blood flow to the injured area. This also facilitates the removal of micro-organisms, foreign debris, bacterial toxins and enzymes by phagocytic cells, complement and antibodies. The coagulation cascade is activated, which isolates the site of infection in a gel-like matrix to protect the host (Dow et al, 1999).

In a chronic wound, however, the continuous presence of virulent micro-organisms leads to a continued inflammatory response, which eventually contributes to host injury. There is persistent production of inflammatory mediators and steady migration of neutrophils, which release cytolytic enzymes and oxygen-free radicals. There is localized thrombosis and the release of vasoconstricting metabolites, which can lead to tissue hypoxia, bringing about further bacterial proliferation and tissue destruction (Dow et al, 1999).

The presence of bacteria in a chronic wound does not necessarily indicate that infection has occurred or that it will lead to the impairment of wound healing (Cooper and Lawrence, 1996). Micro-organisms are present in all chronic wounds and low levels of certain bacteria can actually facilitate healing (De Haan et al, 1974). Bacteria produce proteolytic enzymes, such as hyaluronidase, which contribute to wound debridement and stimulate neutrophils to release proteases (Stone, 1980).

Bacterial burden

When using quantitative bacteriology, infection has been associated with $>10^5$ colony-forming organisms of bacteria per gram of tissue (Gardner et al, 2001). A semi-quantitative swab will provide information on the predominant organisms present, and gives an indication of their density. There remains controversy over the exact technique for taking a wound swab. It is generally recommended that the wound bed be irrigated with saline to remove superficial colonizers, followed by debridement (Sibbald et al, 2003). A dry swab can then be rolled across the exposed bed (Schultz et al, 2003). The swab is inoculated onto solid media and streaked into four quadrants. A rate of 4^+ growth or growth in the fourth quadrant (>30 colonies) corresponds to approximately 10^5 or greater organisms per gram of tissue as measured by quantitative biopsy. This technique samples a large area of the wound surface, but may also lead to an increased number of false-positive results (Schultz et al, 2003).

Bowler (2003) has cast doubt on the merits of quantitative bacteriology as a means of diagnosing wound infection, as infection is dependent on the relationship between the offending micro-organism and the host, and not just on the numbers of bacteria that are present. However, infection may be diagnosed clinically by noting the signs of infection that are present. These signs were initially collated by Cutting and Harding (1994) and then modified by Cutting and White (1994). Subsequently, Cutting et al (2005) have identified infection criteria relevant to six different wound types.

Bacterial involvement in wounds can be divided into four levels, as listed in *Table 11.4*.

In cases of critical colonization, interaction between micro-organisms and host may be of such a nature that a traditional host response is not elicited, and the only sign may be that of delayed healing. A consensus on the features of critical colonization has yet to be reached.

An increased serous exudate may be accompanied by friable granulation tissue that bleeds easily. This granulation tissue may be exuberant and bright red. Bacteria can stimulate angiogenesis, leading to increased vascularity, an abnormal bright red colour and a friable corrupt matrix. When a dressing is removed, the wound surface may bleed easily. An unpleasant or putrid odour may also be accompanied by new areas of necrosis or breakdown in the wound base (Sibbald et al, 2000).

Treatment for infection/inflammation

Treatment should first of all focus on optimizing host resistance, and underlying conditions that reduce immunity should be addressed. Systemic

Table 11.4: Bacterial involvement in wounds

- Wound contamination — The presence of non-replicating micro-organisms, such as soil organisms, in the wound

- Wound colonization — The presence of replicating micro-organisms that are not causing injury to the host. This includes skin commensals, such as *Staphylococcus epidermidis* and *Corynebacterium spp.*, which in most circumstances have been shown to increase the rate of wound healing

- Critical colonization (White et al, 2005) — Bacteria cause a delay in wound healing without frank infection

- Wound infection

From Schultz et al (2003)

antibiotics are not necessarily the most appropriate way of reducing bacterial burden in wounds, particularly because of the threat of increasing bacterial resistance, and should be used where infection cannot be managed with local therapy (Schultz et al, 2003). Other methods may be more suitable and should be considered first: debridement to remove devitalized tissue; wound cleaning; and use of topical antimicrobials, such as silver dressings.

There is renewed interest in the selective use of topical antimicrobials as bacteria become more resistant to antibiotics. Studies show that some iodine and silver preparations have bacteriocidal effects even against multi-resistant organisms such as methicillin-resistant *Staphylococcus aureus* (MRSA) (Lawrence, 1998; Sibbald et al, 2001). Honey also appears to possess potent anti-bacterial properties (Cooper, 2005).

Systemic antibiotic therapy

This should be used in all chronic wounds where there is active infection beyond the level that can be managed with local wound therapy (Sibbald et al, 2003). Systemic signs of infection, such as fever, life-threatening infection, spreading cellulitis and underlying deep structure infections, indicate the use of systemic therapy. However, infected, exudative wounds do not respond well to the use of occlusive dressings and can lead to rapid wound deterioration. In these cases, it is more appropriate to follow debridement with calcium alginate dressings, foams and hydrofibres (Schultz et al, 2003).

M for moisture: restoring moisture balance

Moisture balance needs to be restored at the wound bed to prevent desiccation and maceration. The clinician needs to assess the wound and intervene using the TIME table:

- Clinical sign or symptom — desiccation or excess fluid
- Underlying problem — desiccation slows epithelial migration while excess fluid causes maceration and promotes a hostile biochemical environment, which traps growth factors
- Intervention — appropriate dressings, compression therapy, vacuum-assisted closure (VAC).

In acute wounds, a moist wound environment has been shown to accelerate wound healing by up to 50% compared with exposure to air (Winter, 1962). Wounds that are allowed to dry develop a hard crust, and the underlying collagen matrix and surrounding tissue at the wound edge become desiccated. Keratinocytes must burrow beneath the surface of the crust and matrix if re-epithelialization is to occur as they can only migrate over viable, nutrient-rich tissue and intact extracellular matrix (Schultz et al, 2003). A moist environment physiologically favours migration and matrix formation, and accelerates healing of wounds by promoting autolytic debridement. A wound that is too moist can cause maceration of the surrounding skin. Successful exudate management is about achieving a balance within a fluid environment (Bishop et al, 2003).

Wound with excessive moisture

Numerous clinical trials have demonstrated that wounds treated with occlusive dressings are less likely to become infected than wounds treated with conventional dressings, unless the wound is clinically infected (Hutchinson and Lawrence, 1991). Occlusive dressings are relatively impermeable to exogenous bacteria, encourage the accumulation of natural substances in wound fluid that inhibit bacterial growth and reduce the burden of necrotic tissue in the wound.

However, it is now known that chronic wound fluid contains substances detrimental to cell proliferation (Chen et al, 1999), and the build up of chronic wound fluid must be managed to minimize the negative biochemical factors (*Figure 11.3*).

Indirect approaches to wound exudate management focus on alleviating the underlying cause. Direct wound exudate management involves the use of compression bandages, highly absorbent dressings or vacuum-based, mechanical systems (Ballard and Baxter, 2000). No single dressing matches all the requirements, and the choice of wound dressing at one stage of the wound process may well influence subsequent events in the later phases of healing.

A number of dressings are available to achieve local moisture balance at the wound bed. A guide to selecting the appropriate dressing can be found in *Table 11.5*.

A simple alternative to the use of specialized dressings is to thoroughly clean and irrigate a chronic wound with saline or sterile water, which removes exudate and cellular debris and reduces the bacterial burden of the wound.

Indirect methods of reducing exudate should not be forgotten; although wound fluid may be the result of an elevated bioburden, there are occasions when resolution may be achieved through relief of pressure or elevation of the affected limb.

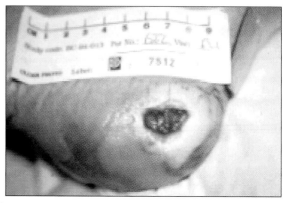

Figure 11.3: Excessive exudate

Table 11.5: Selecting an appropriate dressing to achieve local moisture balance

- Maintains a moist wound environment

- Absorbs excess wound exudates

- Keeps the surrounding skin dry

- Does not require frequent dressing changes

- Decreases the risk of infection by maintaining a seal with the wound

- Is comfortable and acceptable to the patient

Adapted from Schultz et al (2003)

E for edge: non-advancing edge or undermining

When the wound edge fails to migrate or undermining is present (*Figure 11.4*), the clinician needs to reassess the cause and intervene using the TIME table:

- Clinical sign — abnormal epidermal margin or granulation tissue
- Underlying problem — hypertrophic epithelial margin, senescent or altered granulation cells
- Intervention — reassess status of patient and wound; if wound bed is good, consider advanced therapies.

Non-advancing wound edge

Chronic or non-healing ulcers fail to re-epithelialize, and this is usually accompanied by prolonged inflammation (Hasan et al, 1997; Agren et al, 1999; Cook et al, 2000). The epidermis fails to migrate across the wound and there is hyper-proliferation at the wound margins, which interferes with normal cellular migration over the wound bed.

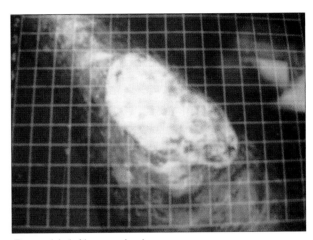

Figure 11.4: Abnormal edge

Perhaps the clearest sign of all that a wound is failing to heal is where the epidermal edge is failing to advance over time towards closure of the wound, as evaluated by the clinician when measuring the wound dimensions. If the margin is undermined, this may be a sign of critical colonization or infection (see earlier), and at a cellular level, lack of epidermal migration could be caused by non-responsive wound cells and abnormalities in protease activity, which degrade extracellular matrix (ECM) as soon as it is formed (Falanga, 2000).

The overall health status of a patient has a significant impact on the wound-healing process. A general medical history, including a medication record, is invaluable in identifying causes that may prevent wound healing. Conditions, such as peripheral vascular disease, diabetes, immobility and malnutrition, must be assessed at the beginning of treatment and corrected as far as possible before local interventions are carried out (Sibbald et al, 2000). If a wound still fails to heal, as demonstrated by a failure to re-epithelialize, it is vital to review these and other factors again and take further intervention if necessary.

Conditions and interventions that are known to delay wound healing include those listed in *Table 11.6*.

Assess tissue perfusion

Wound healing can only take place if there is adequate tissue oxygenation. A well-vascularized wound bed provides nutrients and oxygen to sustain newly-formed granulation tissue and to maintain an active immunological response to microbial invasion. Decreased oxygen levels impair the ability of leucocytes to kill bacteria, lower production of collagen and reduce epithelialization (Schultz et al, 2003).

Wounds of the lower extremities may be particularly affected by poor blood supply. External factors, such as hypothermia, stress or pain, can all increase

Table 11.6: Conditions and interventions that are known to delay wound healing

- Use of systemic steroids

- Use of immunosuppressive drugs

- Use of non-steroidal anti-inflammatories

- Rheumatoid arthritis

- Other autoimmune diseases, such as systemic lupus, uncontrolled vasculitis or pyoderma gangrenosum

- Inadequate or poor nutrition

From Schultz et al (2003)

sympathetic tone and decrease tissue perfusion; smoking reduces microcirculatory flow. In arterial ulcers, macrovascular or microvascular disease leads to tissue ischaemia. A laser Doppler perfusion imaging is a non-invasive method for investigating skin microvasculature (Wardell et al, 1993). If the wound is recurrent, patient education or treatment of an underlying condition may be the critical step in bringing about wound healing. The size, depth and colour of the wound base should be recorded by measurement, such as tracing or photography and recording the colour and type of tissue in the wound bed. This provides a baseline against which healing can be assessed.

The amount and type of exudate (serous, sangous, purulent) should also be assessed; a heavy exudate may indicate uncontrolled oedema or may be an early sign of infection. The points listed in *Table 11.7* need to be noted.

Continuous pain may be because of an underlying cause, local wound irritation or infection. It is important to assess continuous pain to determine if its origin is in the wound or in the surrounding anatomical region (Sibbald et al, 2000).

Continued infection

Host resistance is the single most important determinant of wound infection and should be rigorously assessed whenever a chronic wound fails to heal (Dow et al,

Table 11.7: Wound assessment considerations

- Check wound margin for callus formation, maceration, oedema or erythema

- Check for hyperkeratotic calluses on the plantar aspect of the foot in patients with neuropathy. The callus should be removed to reduce pressure

- White hyperkeratosis of the surrounding skin or ulcer margin and an overhydrated wound surface suggest excess fluid

- Limb oedema or uncorrected pressure may be causes of local oedema

- Maceration may be a sign of infection

- Warm, hot, tender erythema suggests infection

- Discreet erythema with well-demarcated margins indicates contact allergic dermatitis caused by applied dressings or topical treatments

From Schultz et al (2003)

1999). Systemic host resistance can be affected by many variables, some of which may be behavioural leading to non-concordance. In such cases, wound management will involve not only treatment of the wound, but also treatment of the underlying disease. The use of cytotoxic agents and cortiocosteroids can totally mask all signs of local or systemic infection (Schultz et al, 2003).

Host defence mechanisms may be enhanced by a number of methods appropriate to the particular condition of the patient. An infected chronic wound in the presence of critical limb ischaemia may be improved by reconstructive vascular surgery, for example, and bacterial burden may be reduced by measures designed to control blood sugar in the patient with diabetes.

Advanced techniques

The principles of TIME should be used as a checklist to assess that all appropriate interventions have been made (*Table 11.8*).

If this systematic approach produces a well-vascularized, healthy wound bed that still fails to heal, it may be that advanced therapies are necessary to 'kick-start' the process of healing. The patient will need to be referred for specialist advice and advanced therapies.

The following advanced techniques are all effective if applied to a well-prepared wound bed, but can only be carried out by skilled clinicians: autologous skin grafts; grafting using cultured cells/keratinocytes; bioengineered products; allogenic, bilayered tissue; and artificial skin. In

Table 11.8: The principles of TIME that should act as a checklist when assessing that interventions have been made
■ Has all necrotic tissue been debrided?
■ Is there a well-vascularized wound bed?
■ Has infection been brought under control?
■ Is inflammation under control?
■ Has moisture imbalance been corrected?
■ What dressings have been applied?

From Schultz et al (2003)

addition, a number of growth factors have been developed, which are usually supplied in a mesh that is applied to the surface of the wound. Data on the performance of these growth factors has been emerging over the last decade (Schultz et al, 2003):

- Basic fibroblast growth factor — stimulates endothelial cell proliferation and migration
- Transforming growth factor β — stimulates the growth of fibroblasts and keratinocytes as well as the production of extracellular matrix, particularly collagen
- Endothelial growth factor — supports the growth of keratinocytes and assists the migration of keratinocytes, fibroblasts and endothelial cells
- Platelet-derived growth factor — chemotactic for polymorphonuclear cells and macrophages.

Conclusion

Wound bed preparation consists of basic steps that help to stimulate healing. The wound bed preparation process acknowledges that the acute-wound healing models do not apply to chronic wounds, and a systematic approach is needed to address the underlying molecular and cellular imbalance that is usually responsible for non-healing in a chronic wound. The end result may be wound closure, which will eliminate the need for advanced therapies or procedures. If, however, advanced therapies, such as skin grafts or growth factors and skin substitutes, are still required for wound closure, the success of these techniques will be greatly improved if applied to a well-prepared wound bed.

Wound bed preparation provides a rational approach to the management of non-healing wounds, which can be supported with reference to the underlying cellular environment. Wound bed preparation is part of a more systematic and, ultimately, more effective approach to wound management.

This chapter is based on Schultz GS, Sibbald GR, Falanga V et al (2003) Wound bed preparation: a systematic approach to wound management. Wound Repair Regen *11(2): 1–28*

References

Agren MS, Steenfos HH, Dabelsteen S, Hansen JB, Dabelsteen E (1999) Proliferation and mitogenic response to PDGF-BB of fibroblasts isolated from chronic leg ulcers is ulcer-dependent. *J Invest Dermatol* **112:** 463–69

Baharestani M (1999) The clinical relevance of debridement. In: Baharestani M, Goltrup F, Holstein P, Vanscheidt W, eds. *The Clinical Relevance of Debridement.* Springer-Verlag, Berlin, Heidelberg

Ballard K, Baxter H (2000) Developments in wound care for difficult-to-manage wounds. *Br J Nurs* **9:** 405–12

Bishop SM, Walker M, Rogers AA, Chen WY (2003) Importance of moisture balance at the wound-dressing interface. *J Wound Care* **12**(4): 125–8

Bowler PG (2003) The 10^5 bacterial growth guideline: reassessing its clinical relevance in wound healing. *Ostomy Wound Manage* **49**(1): 44–53

Chen WY, Rogers AA, Lydon MJ (1999) Characterization of biologic properties of wound fluid collected during early stages of wound healing. *J Invest Dermatol* **99:** 559–64

Cook H, Davies KJ, Harding KG, Thomas DW (2000) Defective extracellular matrix reorganization by chronic wound fibroblasts is associated with alterations in TIMP-1, TIMP-2 and MMP-2 activity. *J Invest Dermatol* **115:** 225–33

Cooper R (2005) The antimicrobial activity of honey. In: White R, Cooper R, Molan P, eds. *Honey: A Modern Wound Management Product.* Aberdeen Wounds UK, Aberdeen

Cooper RA, Lawrence JC (1996) Micro-organisms and wounds. *J Wound Care* **5**(5): 233–6

Cutting KF, Harding KG (1994) Criteria for identifying wound infection. *J Wound Care* **3**(4): 198–201

Cutting KF, White RJ (2005) Criteria for identifying wound infection — revisited. *Ostomy Wound Manage* **51**(1): 28–34

Cutting KF, White RJ, Mahoney P, Harding KG (2005) Clinical identification of wound infection: a Delphi approach. In: *Identifying Criteria for Wound Infection.* Position statement. EWMA/MEP, London

De Haan BB, Ellis H, Wilkes M (1974) The role of infection in wound healing. *Surg Gynecol Obstet* **138:** 697–700

Dealey C (2002) *The Care of Wounds: a Guide for Nurses.* Blackwell Science, Oxford

Dow G, Browne A, Sibbald RG (1999) Infection in chronic wounds: controversies in diagnosis and treatment. *Ostomy Wound Manage* **45:** 23–40

Ennis WJ, Meneses P (2000) Wound healing at the local level. The stunned wound. *Ostomy Wound Manage* **46:** 39S–48S

Fairbairn K, Grier J, Hunter J, Preece J (2002) A sharp debridement procedure devised by specialist nurses. *J Wound Care* **11**(10): 371–5

Falanga V (2000) Classifications for wound bed preparation and stimulation of chronic wounds. *Wound Repair Regen* **8:** 347–52

Falanga V (2002) Wound bed preparation and the role of enzymes: a case for multiple actions of therapeutic agents. *Wounds* **4**(2): 47–57

Falanga V, Grinnell F, Gilchrist B, Maddox YT, Moshell A (1994) Workshop on the pathogenesis of chronic wounds. *J Invest Dermatol* **102**(1): 125–7

Flanagan M (1997) *Wound Management.* Churchill Livingstone, London

Gardner SE, Frantz RA, Doebbeling BN (2001) The validity of the clinical signs and symptoms used to identify localized chronic wound infection. *Wound Repair Regen* **9:** 178–86

Gray D, White R, Cooper P, Kingsley A (2005) Understanding Applied Wound Management. *Wounds UK* **1**(2): 4–8

Hasan A, Murata H, Falabella A, Ochoa S, Zhou L, Badiava E, Falanga V (1997) Dermal fibroblasts from venous ulcers are unresponsive to action of transforming growth factor-beta I. *J Dermatol Sci* **16:** 59–66

Hutchinson JJ, Lawrence JC (1991) Wound infection under occlusive dressings. *J Hosp Infect* **17:** 83–94

Kerstein MD (1997) The scientific basis of healing. *Adv Wound Care* **10:** 30–6

Lawrence JC (1998) The use of iodine as an antiseptic. *J Wound Care* **7**(8): 421–5

O'Brien M (2002) Exploring methods of wound debridement. *Br J Community Nurs* **7**(12) (Suppl): 10–18

Schultz G, Sibbald G, Falanga V et al (2003) Wound bed preparation: a systematic approach to wound management. *Wound Repair Regen* **11**(2): 1–28

Sibbald RG, Williamson D, Orsted HL, Campbell K, Keast D, Krasner D, Sibbald D (2000) Preparing the wound bed — debridement, bacterial balance and moisture balance. *Ostomy Wound Manage* **46:** 14–35

Sibbald RG, Browne AC, Coutts P, Queen D (2001) Screening evaluation of an ionized nanocrystalline silver dressing in chronic wound care. *Ostomy Wound Manage* **47:** 38–43

Sibbald RG, Orsted H, Schyltz G, Coutts RN, Keast MD (2003) Preparing the wound bed: focus on infection and inflammation. *Ostomy Wound Manage* **49**(11): 24–51

Steed DL, Donohoe D, Webster MW, Lindsley L (1996) Effect of extensive debridement and treatment on the healing of diabetic foot ulcers. *J Am Coll Surg* **183:** 61–4

Stone LL (1980) Bacterial debridement of the burn eschar: the *in-vivo* activity of selected organisms. *J Surg Res* **29:** 83–92

Tortora GJ, Grabowski SR (2000) *Principles of Anatomy and Physiology.* 9th edn. John Wiley, New York

Vowden K, Vowden P (1999) Wound debridement: 1. *J Wound Care* 8(5): 237–40

Wardell K, Jakobsson A, Nilsson GE (1993) Laser Doppler perfusion imaging by dynamic light scattering. *IEEE Trans Biomed Eng* **40:** 309–16

White RJ, Cutting KF, Kingsley A (2005) Critical colonisation: clinical reality or myth? *Wounds UK* **1**(1): 94–5

Winter GD (1962) Formation of the scab and the rate of epithelialisation of superficial wounds in the skin of the young domestic pig. *Nature* **193:** 293–4

Chapter 12

Wound management: the considerations involved in dressing selection

Kathryn Vowden

Dressing selection requires a careful assessment of the patient and wound, the development of an individualized clinical management plan and an evaluation of treatment effectiveness. Dressings have specific functions; appropriate product selection can aid healing and improve outcome and therefore patients' quality of life by minimizing their symptoms. TELER (treatment evaluation by Le Roux's method) provides an effective way of monitoring care, both from the health professional's and the patient's perspective, and is a useful tool to assess progress.

Effective wound care is dependent on accurate assessment, investigations, informed diagnosis and appropriate product selection. Previous research into the prescribing of dressings has served to emphasize the random nature of product selection that can occur in wound management (Bux and Malhi, 1996; Barlow, 1999a,b).

The cost of prescribing wound care products in general practice in 2003 exceeded £138 million (Department of Health (DoH), 2004). A report from the National Prescribing Centre (NPC) indicated that there was a lack of randomized, controlled trials to assess the effectiveness of wound care products. It also highlighted that there was evidence that non-effective treatments were being prescribed (DoH, 1999). In an attempt to address some of these problems, both national guidelines (Royal College of Nursing (RCN), 1998; National Institute for Clinical Excellence (NICE), 2001) and local policy and formularies have been developed to aid product selection and reduce cost by improving effectiveness. The seven principles of good prescribing (NPC, 1999) provide a framework within which wound care can be approached.

Dressings should never be used in isolation, but should function as part of an overall clinical management plan that addresses issues raised in the holistic assessment of the patient. This will include the control of risk factors for delayed healing, the management of any underlying disease, protection of the wound and patient from further trauma, the state of the surrounding skin, the management of infection and pain and the most appropriate method of dressing fixation.

Information to aid prescribing

Each clinical situation provides a unique set of factors that impact on dressing selection and performance, and which vary over time. Individual dressing selection should be based on a combination of available clinical and laboratory data relating to the underlying pathological condition being treated, the known physical and biochemical properties of the wound care product selected, and the patient's known sensitivities, requirements and expectations. Once a product or combination of products is selected, the effectiveness of care must be continually evaluated and the outcome assessed and used to inform future product selection. It is the responsibility of the prescriber to re-evaluate dressing performance in each clinical situation and to use the information to modify an individual's treatment plan and to inform future formulary design. These rules conform to the seven principles of good prescribing (NPC, 1999).

Information on selection of dressings

Independent information on individual dressings is available online at *World Wide Wounds* (www.worldwidewounds.com/Common/ProductDatacards.html) and *Dressings.org* (www.dressings.org). Details can also be obtained from the *British National Formulary* (Joint Formulary Committee, 2004). The information contained in these sources, however, is based on dressing types rather than function, which may be more useful when selecting individual products.

Laboratory-based studies describe the physical characteristics of products but do not necessarily inform on their performance in the clinical situation. Data is available on:

- Absorbency (Thomas and Fram, 2001)
- Vapour permeability (Erasmus and Jonkman, 1989)
- Odour containment (Thomas et al, 1998)

- Bacterial control (Thomas and McCubbin, 2003)
- Other measurable factors, such as adhesion, strength and elasticity (Queen et al, 1987; Lin et al, 2001; Thomas, 2003a).

Careful review of these and other papers show that the testing process does not always relate to the variety of dressing demands that occur in 'real world' clinical situations, and therefore further information is required.

Although clinical trials do provide some information that is useful to health practitioners, there remains a dearth of detailed, randomized, comparative studies on the relative effectiveness of dressings, and this is reflected in reports from NICE (2001) and from the Cochrane Wounds Group (*Table 12.1*).

Table 12.1: The Cochrane Wounds Group — internet references
www.york.ac.uk/healthsciences/gsp/themes/woundcare/Wounds/index.htm
Abstracts of Cochrane Reviews relating to wound care:
www.update-software.com/abstracts/WOUNDSAbstractIndex.htm

The nature of clinical trials requires that inclusion and exclusion criteria are satisfied. For this reason, most clinical trials do not address dressing performance in complex clinical situations, particularly where product combinations are required such as when absorptive dressings are used under compression bandages. These studies also tend to focus on healing as the study endpoint, rather than short-term goals such as exudate containment, pain relief or debridement.

There are few studies that include patients with multiple diseases which, according to Schofield et al (2003), are a significant problem in the elderly. They demonstrated in their leg ulcer population that 57% had four or more other diagnoses. These diseases may impact on treatment or healing outcome and are important considerations when selecting wound treatment. In addition, studies rarely look at 'never'-to-heal wounds, such as malignant ulceration, where symptomatic control is the primary aim (Grocott, 1998, 2000).

In an attempt to rationalize the process of wound management and to enable the consideration of appropriate management strategies, the concept of wound bed preparation was conceived (Falanga, 2000; Vowden and Vowden, 2002). This concept continues to evolve and has recently been summarized in the acronym TIME (tissue management; inflammation and infection; moisture balance; and epithelial edge advancement) (Schultz et al, 2003). TIME has been developed to reflect specific dressing selection guidelines for different wound types (European Wound Management Association, 2004). It can be used as a basis for dressing selection based on the functional outcome required, including:

- Debridement
- Bacterial management
- Exudate management
- Edge stimulation and healing.

Dressing performance and patient evaluation

Four of the seven principles of good prescribing comprise concordance, review of progress, documentation and reflection. In terms of wound care, dressing choice, performance and patient progress are based around three additional interactive factors:

- The product
- The health professional
- The patient.

From the patient's perspective, dressing performance can be measured in terms of:

- Fit — does the product conform to and fit the wound and body surface?
- Feel — is the product comfortable to apply, wear and remove?
- Form — is the product available in a suitable range of sizes and functions for effective clinical use?
- Function — does the product perform the function for which it was designed?

Dressing choice by the health professional is informed by the state of the wound, the underlying wound aetiology, the state of the patient, the expected outcome for the intervention (debridement, infection control and exudate management), and product availability and cost. Cost, however, must be measured in terms of overall effectiveness and not individual product costs (Harding et al, 2000; Franks, 2001). There is a vast array of dressing products on the market. Each dressing type has a broad functional classification, which is illustrated in *Figure 12.1*.

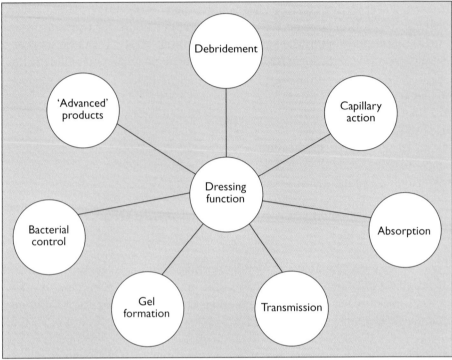

Figure 12.1: Diagrammatic representation of available choices in dressing selection based on dressing function

Debridement

There are a number of products where debridement is the primary function. These range from dressings that rehydrate necrotic tissue and eschar, to more active treatments such as larval therapy (Vowden and Vowden, 1999a,b). The choice of product is based on the needs of the patient, the goals, the timescale in which to achieve the goal safely, and factors relating to the patient assessment and disease process.

Capillary action

These types of dressings are usually multi-layered. The inner, non-adherent layer conducts the fluid vertically, while subsequent layers hold and dissipate the fluid throughout the outer component of the dressing, conducting fluid away from the wound surface. They have been shown to be effective in moderate- to high-volume and low- to moderate-viscosity exudating wounds (Russell et al, 2001; Deeth, 2002). However, a study on a capillary dressing conducted by Reynolds et al (2004) demonstrated that although these dressings appeared effective in unblinded assessment, they failed to show benefit in blinded assessment.

Cadexomer beads can function in a similar way; fluid is taken into the beads along an osmotic gradient and away the from the wound surface (Marzin, 1993). In some cadexomer products, iodine is released into the wound environment producing a bactericidal effect (Hansson, 1998). These dressings may also assist in the debridement process (Lisle, 2002).

Absorptive dressings

Absorptive dressings consist of foam or a pad with a primary non-adherent wound contact layer. They can handle moderate to high volumes of fluid, but do not manage high-viscosity exudate well. The dressings do not rehydrate necrotic tissue but do assist autolytic debridement by maintaining a moist environment at the wound bed, while reducing the risk of wound margin maceration. The foam dressings fall into two basic categories: a simple foam dressing; and a foam dressing that has a vapour-permeable film backing to allow evaporation of fluid from the dressing surface. Absorptive dressings have been shown to be effective in a number of wound types (Collier, 1992; Thomas, 1997a,b; Taylor et al, 1999), but the dressing's absorptive capacity can be compromised under pressure, such as when used with high-compression bandaging. Foam dressings tend not to conform well and are in general difficult to use with cavity wounds unless specifically designed to do so (Berry et al, 1996).

Transmission

Transmission dressings manage fluid load by allowing the evaporation of components such as water vapour from the dressing surface. Fluid loss is recorded as the dressing moisture vapour transmission rate (MVTR). Most laboratory work in this field has been in the assessment of film dressings (Thomas, 1996; Thomas et al, 1997a,b). The selective release of water vapour can result in a concentration of the other, potentially damaging, components within the exudate, some of which may be held at the wound surface.

Some dressings combine the action of transmission and absorbency into a single composite dressing. This increases the volume of exudate these dressings can handle, and holds the 'concentrated' exudate within the absorbent layer. In general, these dressings are most suitable for acute, low to moderate-volume, low-viscosity and exudating wounds, although they have been shown to be of value in high-volume, low-viscosity exudating malignant wounds.

Gel formation

One component of the dressing (frequently a hydrocolloid, hydrogel, alginate or hydrofibre) takes up fluid to form a gel and holds it in the dressing but in contact with the wound surface, maintaining a moist wound environment and facilitating autolytic debridement. The time taken for a gel to form varies between products. Depending on the formulation, hydrocolloids and hydrogels can either absorb exudate or rehydrate a wound and are most suitable for wounds with a low- to moderate-volume or moderate- to high-viscosity exudate.

Alginate (Stewart, 2002) and hydrofibre dressings are suitable for moderate- to high-volume, moderate- to high-viscosity exudates. Hydrofibres have been shown to be effective in heavily exudating, acute (Foster and Moore, 1997; Robinson, 2000) and chronic wounds (Armstrong and Ruckley, 1997), and their relatively pain-free removal can be an advantage (Moore and Foster, 2000). Depending on the formulation of the product, other elements in the exudate such as bacteria or matrix metaloproteinases may be absorbed or modified (Stewart, 2002). Hydrocolloids and hydrogels are most suitable for wounds with a low- to moderate-volume exudate.

Bacterial control

Products containing iodine (Hunt and Middlekoop, 1995; Gilchrist, 1997) and silver can, through their antiseptic or antimicrobial action, reduce the bacterial load (Stewart, 2002) and may reduce exudate levels. Such dressings are suitable for moderately to heavily exudating (high volume and viscosity) wounds, with evidence of heavy bacterial colonization or overt infection.

The antimicrobial effects of silver-containing dressings have been reviewed by Thomas and McCubbin (2003). The wider role of silver has been reviewed by several authors (Demling and DeSanti, 2001; Lansdown,

2002a,b). In a comparative study of several silver-containing dressings, Lansdown et al (2005) concluded that silver dressings were safe for use in chronic wound therapy, but that further studies are needed to examine the potential for silver resistance, an area discussed further by Percival et al (2005).

The role of iodine and its impact on wound physiology has been discussed by Hunt and Middlekoop (1995), and similar conclusions have been reached about their safety and efficacy in chronic wound care. These dressings often have an additional debriding action, and function well when used in combination with compression therapy in the management of the ulcerated, oedematous limb.

The slow release of antimicrobials from some products reduces the need for frequent dressing changes and has, in the case of silver-containing dressings, been suggested to act as a barrier to the transmission of methicillin-resistant *Staphylococcus aureus* (MRSA) (Strohal et al, 2005). An alternative approach to bacterial load management is the use of honey, which has been demonstrated to be effective in the management of wound infection (Kingsley, 2001; Cooper, 2005) and has a debriding action.

Advanced products

This is a generic grouping of products that stimulate the wound bed and which include Promogran, hyaluronic acid, growth factors and vacuum-assisted closure (VAC) therapy, which uses negative pressure to both remove the exudate and improve the local wound environment, enhancing healing. Topical negative-pressure (TNP) devices, which are suitable for high-volume and low- to high-viscosity exudate wounds, have been suggested to reduce bacterial load (Morykwas et al, 1997) and to remove bacterial toxins, matrix metaloproteinases and other toxic chemicals from the wound environment, facilitating debridement; manipulation and control of wound pH may enhance healing by modifying protease activity (Greener et al, 2005).

There is increasing interest in the field of tissue engineering and the use of human tissue equivalents in chronic wound care. A range of products are available that aim to provide either an extracellular matrix or cellular components of dermis or skin, and which in turn act as a source of growth factors. However, careful consideration should be given before using advanced therapies as these products are more costly.

Flanagan (2001) suggests that before using advanced wound care products the following questions should be considered:

- Has the patient been thoroughly assessed?
- Is the treatment specifically indicated?
- What potential benefits will the use of this therapy bring?
- Have all other alternatives been considered?

Bandage considerations and selection

Bandages serve three basic functions: retention of dressings, support and compression. Thomas has conducted a number of reviews of bandage type and function (Thomas, 1990; Thomas, 1997b; Thomas and Nelson, 1998; Thomas, 2003), and these papers provide the knowledge to underpin clinical use of the wide variety of products available. The most specific therapeutic use of bandages is to provide compression, particularly in the management of venous ulceration.

The role of, and rationale for, compression therapy in the management of venous disease is well researched and has been summarized in an *Effective Health Care Bulletin* (NHS Centre for Reviews and Dissemination, 1997) and in a *Cochrane Review* (Cullum et al, 2001). International guidelines for compression therapy exist (Stacey et al, 2002), and these have formed the basis for a recent position paper from the European Wound Management Association (2003). All these papers comment on the importance of assessment, and in particular the measurement of the ankle brachial pressure index before the application of compression therapy.

On the current available evidence there appears to be little difference in the effectiveness of the type of high-compression bandage system used. However, good bandaging technique is vital if maximum effect and safety are to be assured. To assist application, some bandages include markings to aid application at the correct extension. RCN guidelines (1998) advise that the compression is only applied by a suitably trained health professional, to ensure the effectiveness and safety of this treatment.

Evaluating treatment and dressings

No single measure of dressing or bandage performance is appropriate, given the wide range of products available and the varied functions they perform. Dressing effectiveness has to be measured against a number of standards, which include the patient's perception of care and not just the views of health professionals or manufacturers.

The Woundcare Research for Appropriate Products (WRAP) group has recently reported on the validation of TELER (treatment evaluation by Le Roux's method) in the assessment of dressing performance (Browne et al, 2004). The system, which uses a series of indicators to measure significant clinical change and a statistical method of measurement, provides a note-taking system that records the relationship between the care provided, including dressing and nursing performance, and outcomes. Care evaluation includes details on:

■ The state of the surrounding skin
■ Wound management and dressing performance
■ The patient's experience
■ Symptom control.

The system is based on a series of assumptions, which can be summarized as:

■ Effective treatment is patient-centred
■ Effective treatment is grounded in theory
■ The essential purpose of treatment is to induce or prevent change
■ Change or lack of change occurs in clinically significant steps over clinically significant periods of time
■ Change or lack of change, which is unlikely to have occurred by chance, was induced
■ The effects of clinically significant change are not necessarily measurable on an interval or ratio scale, but they are observable.

Table 12.2: TELER: surrounding skin — white maceration from exudate

Code		
5	No white maceration from exudate	
4	Skin has a few (less than 4) isolated, white, dull patches	
3	Skin has multiple (more than 4) isolated, white, dull patches	
2	Skin has multiple, white, dull patches that are joining together	
1	The skin is entirely white and dull	
0	The white, dull epidermal skin has separated, exposing the dermis	

Table 12.3: TELER: dressing performance (bandaging) — exudate leaking (bandaging)

Code		
	5	Dressing marked, bandage unmarked
	4	Dressing wet, bandage unmarked
	3	Dressing sodden, bandage marked
	2	Dressing and bandage sodden
	1	Bandage sodden and shoes marked
	0	Bandage and shoes sodden

Table 12.4: TELER: patient experience — impact of odour

Components	a. Worried others will notice odour
	b. Aware of an odour
	c. Using deodorizers or perfume
	d. Affects socialization
	e. Other — please state

Code		
	5	Not experiencing any components
	4	Experiencing 1 component
	3	Experiencing 2 components
	2	Experiencing 3 components
	1	Experiencing 4 components
	0	Experiencing 5 components

Table 12.5: TELER: symptom control — odour

Code		
	5	No odour
	4	Odour is detected on removal of the dressing
	3	Odour is evident on exposure of the dressing
	2	Odour is evident at arms length from the patient
	1	Odour is evident on entering the room
	0	Odour is evident on entering house/ward/clinic

Tables 12.2–12.5 give examples of the coded scoring system, each clinical indicator having six clinically significant reference points (codes 0–5).

The TELER indicators act as an ordinal measuring scale, which can be used to monitor change over time. These data can then be translated into measures of clinical effectiveness, which involves the patient in his/her treatment and the outcome measure. The criteria measured are the:

- Deficit index — a measure of the effect of the problems as they present
- Improvement index — monitors the scale of improvement relative to the deficit
- Maintenance index — shows the patient's condition relative to the potential for deterioration
- Effectiveness of care index — shows the extent to which treatment and care are managed in the therapeutic process
- Health gain index — standardized index that summarizes the above.

By following changes over time, a graphic representation of progress in care and outcome and dressing performance can be made (*Figure 12.2*). This approach allows a clear distinction between the contributions of clinical practice and wound dressing performance, and allows 'failures' to be correctly attributed to the appropriate area of care (clinical care, decision making, dressing product, patient factors and medical problems). Such a system of evaluation is necessary if effective dressing usage is to be achieved, and it provides a means for reflective practice in relation to dressing use and care provision.

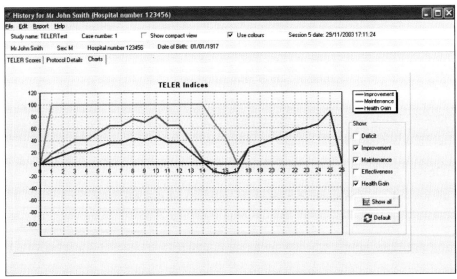

Figure 12.2: Graphic representation of the maintenance index, health gain index and improvement index during treatment for a simulated patient

Conclusions

Appropriate dressing selection requires an in-depth assessment of the patient and the wound, knowledge of the physical and functional properties of the products to be used and a defined and measurable aim for the intervention. The assessment should identify the aetiology of the wound, risk factors for delayed healing and associated medical conditions, potential problems (e.g. allergy and sensitivity), as well as recording the physical characteristics of the wound (size, edge, depth, exudate level, pain and wound bed and bacterial load status). Patient involvement in the process of treatment planning is necessary to assist concordance, and a system of documentation must be in place to record the treatment aims and outcomes in terms of the aims of both health professional and patient.

References

Armstrong SH, Ruckley CV (1997) Use of a fibrous dressing in exuding leg ulcers. *J Wound Care* **6**(7): 322–4

Barlow J (1999a) Prescribing for leg ulcers in general practice: Part 1. *J Wound Care* **8**(7): 369–71

Barlow J (1999b) Prescribing for leg ulcers in general practice: Part 2. *J Wound Care* **8**(8): 390–4

Berry DP, Bale S, Harding KG (1996) Dressings for treating cavity wounds. *J Wound Care* **5**: 10–17

Browne N, Grocott P, Cowley S et al (2004) Woundcare Research for Appropriate Products (WRAP): validation of the TELER method involving users. *Int J Nurs Stud* **41**(5): 559–71

Bux M, Malhi JS (1996) Assessing the use of dressings in practice. *J Wound Care* **5**(7): 305–8

Collier J (1992) A moist, odour-free environment. A multicentred trial of a foamed gel and a hydrocolloid dressing. *Prof Nurse* **7**(12): 804–8

Cooper R (2005) The antimicrobial activity of honey. In: White R, Cooper R, Molan P, eds. *Honey: A Modern Wound Management Product*. Wounds UK Ltd, Aberdeen: 24–32

Cullum NA, Nelson EA, Fletcher AW, Sheldon TA (2001) Compression for venous leg ulcers. *Cochrane Database Syst Rev* (2). Update Software, Oxford

Deeth M (2002) Review of an independent audit into the clinical efficacy of VACUTEX. *Br J Nurs* **11**(12 Suppl): S60–6

Demling RH, DeSanti L (2001) The role of silver technology in wound healing, part 1: effect of silver on wound management. *Wounds: A Compendium of Clinical Research and Practice* **13**(1 (Supplement A)): 4–15

Department of Health (1999) *Prescription Cost Analysis: England 1999.* DoH, London

Department of Health (2004) *Prescription Cost Analysis: England 2003.* DoH, London

Erasmus ME, Jonkman MF (1989) Water vapour permeance: a meaningful measure for water vapour permeability of wound coverings. *Burns* **15**(6): 371–5

European Wound Management Association (2003) *Understanding Compression Therapy.* Position statement. Spring 2003. EWMA/MEP, London

European Wound Management Association (2004) *Wound Bed Preparation in Practice.* Position statement. Spring 2004. EWMA/MEP, London

Falanga V (2000) Classifications for wound bed preparation and stimulation of chronic wounds. *Wound Repair Regen* **8**(5): 347–52

Flanagan M (2001) Dedicated followers of fashion. *Nurs Times* **97**(9): 1

Foster L, Moore P (1997) The application of a cellulose-based fibre dressing in surgical wounds. *J Wound Care* **6**(10): 469–73

Franks P (2001) What do we mean by cost effective wound care? *Eur Wound Manage Assoc J* **1**(1): 25–7

Gilchrist B (1997) Should iodine be reconsidered in wound management? European Tissue Repair Society. *J Wound Care* **6**(3): 148–50

Greener B, Hughes AA, Bannister NP, Douglass J (2005) Proteases and pH in chronic wounds. *J Wound Care* **14:** 59–61

Grocott P (1998) Exudate management in fungating wounds. *J Wound Care* **7**(9): 445–8

Grocott P (2000) The palliative management of fungating malignant wounds. *J Wound Care* **9**(1): 4–9

Hansson C (1998) The effects of cadexomer iodine paste in the treatment of venous leg ulcers compared with hydrocolloid dressing and paraffin gauze dressing. Cadexomer Iodine Study Group. *Int J Dermatol* **37**(5): 390–6

Harding K, Cutting K, Price P (2000) The cost-effectiveness of wound management protocols of care. *Br J Nurs* **9**(19 Suppl): S6–S10

Hunt T, Middlekoop E, eds (1995) *Iodine and Wound Physiology: A Symposium.* Proceedings of 5th Annual Meeting of the European Tissue Repair Society. European Tissue Repair Society, Padua, Italy

Joint Formulary Committee (2004) *British National Formulary 47.* March. British Medical Association and Royal Pharmaceutical Society of Great Britain, London

Kingsley A (2001) The use of honey in the treatment of infected wounds: case studies. *Br J Nurs* **10:** S13–6, S18, S20

Lansdown AB (2002a) Silver 1: its antibacterial properties and mechanism of action. *J Wound Care* **11**(4): 125–30

Lansdown AB (2002b) Silver 2: toxicity in mammals and how its products aid wound repair. *J Wound Care* **11**(5): 173–7

Lansdown AB, Williams A, Chandler S, Benfield S (2005) Silver absorption and antibacterial efficacy of silver dressings. *J Wound Care* **14:** 155–60

Lin SY, Chen KS, Run-Chu L (2001) Design and evaluation of drug-loaded wound dressing having thermoresponsive, adhesive, absorptive and easy peeling properties. *Biomaterials* **22**(22): 2999–3004

Lisle J (2002) Debridement of necrotic tissue and eschar using a capillary dressing and semi-permeable film dressing. *Br J Community Nurs* **7**(9 Suppl): 29–34

Marzin L (1993) Comparing dextranomer absorbant pads and dextanomer paste in the treatment of venous leg ulcers. *J Wound Care* **2**(2): 80–3

Moore PJ, Foster L (2000) Cost benefits of two dressings in the management of surgical wounds. *Br J Nurs* **9**(17): 1128–32

Morykwas MJ, Argenta LC, Shelton-Brown EI, McGuirt W (1997) Vacuum-assisted closure: a new method for wound control and treatment: animal studies and basic foundation. *Ann Plast Surg* **38**(6): 553–62

National Institute for Clinical Excellence (2001) *Guidance on the Use of Debriding Agents and Specialist Wound Care Clinics for Difficult to Heal Surgical Wounds.* NICE. Available at www.nice.org.uk/page.aspx?o=17267 (accessed 17 June 2004)

National Prescribing Centre (1999) Signposts for prescribing nurses — general principles of good prescribing. *Prescribing Nurse Bulletin* **1**(1): 1–4

NHS Centre for Reviews and Dissemination (1997) Compression therapy for venous leg ulcers. Effective Health Care Bulletin. NHSCRD, York. www.york.ac.uk/inst/crd/ehc34.pdf (accessed 17 June 2004)

Percival SL, Bowler PG, Russell D (2005) Bacterial resistance to silver in wound care. *J Hosp Infect* **60:** 1–7

Queen D, Evans JH, Gaylor JD, Courtney JM, Reid WH (1987) An *in-vitro* assessment of wound dressing conformability. *Biomaterials* **8**(5): 372–6

Reynolds T, Russell L, Deeth M, Jones H, Birchall L (2004) A randomised controlled trial comparing Drawtex with standard dressings for exuding wounds. *J Wound Care* **13:** 71–4

Royal College of Nursing (1998) *Clinical Practice Guidelines: The Management of Patients with Venous Leg Ucers.* RCN, London. www.rcn.org.uk/publications/pdf/guidelines/venous_leg_ulcers.pdf (accessed 17 June 2004)

Robinson BJ (2000) The use of a hydrofibre dressing in wound management. *J Wound Care* **9**(1): 32–4

Russell L, Deeth M, Jones HM, Reynolds T (2001) VACUTEX capillary action dressing: a multicentre, randomized trial. *Br J Nurs* **10**(11 Suppl): S66–70

Schofield M, Aziz M, Bliss MR, Bull RH (2003) Medical pathology in patients with leg ulcers: a study carried out in a leg ulcer clinic in a day hospital for the elderly. *J Tissue Viability* **13**(1): 17–22

Schultz GS, Sibbald RG, Falanga V et al (2003) Wound bed preparation: a systematic approach to wound management. *Wound Repair Regen* **11**(Suppl 1): S1–S28

Stacey MC, Falanga V, Marston W et al (2002) The use of compression therapy in the treatment of venous leg ulcers. *Eur Wound Manage Assoc J* **2**(1): 9–13

Stewart J (2002) Next generation products for wound management. *World Wide Wounds.* November. Available: www.worldwidewounds.com/2003/april/Stewart/Next-Generation-Products.html (accessed 17 June 2004)

Strohal R, Schelling M, Takacs M, Jurecka W, Gruber U, Offner F (2005) Nanocrystalline silver dressings as an efficient anti-MRSA barrier: a new solution to an increasing problem. *J Hosp Infect* **60:** 226-30

Taylor A, Lane C, Walsh J, Whittaker S, Ballard K, Young SR (1999) A non-comparative multi-centre clinical evaluation of a new hydropolymer adhesive dressing. *J Wound Care* **8**(10): 489–92

Thomas S (1990) Bandages and bandaging: the science behind the art. *Care Science and Practice* **8**(2): 56–60

Thomas S (1996) Vapour-permeable film dressings. *J Wound Care* **5**(6): 271–4

Thomas S (1997a) Assessment and management of wound exudate. *J Wound Care* **6**(7): 327–30

Thomas S (1997b) Compression bandaging in the treatment of venous leg ulcers. *World Wide Wounds.* September. Available: www.worldwidewounds.com/1997/september/Thomas-Bandaging/bandage-paper.html (accessed 17 June 2004)

Thomas S (2003a) Atraumatic dressings. *World Wide Wounds.* Available: www.worldwidewounds.com/2003/january/Thomas/Atraumatic-Dressings.html (accessed 28 June 2004)

Thomas S (2003b) The use of the Laplace equation in the calculation of sub-bandage pressure. *World Wide Wounds.* June. Available: www.worldwidewounds.com/2003/june/Thomas/Laplace-Bandages.html (accessed 17 June 2004)

Thomas S, Fisher B, Fram PJ, Waring MJ (1998) Odour-absorbing dressings. *J Wound Care* **7**(5): 246–50

Thomas S, Nelson E (1998) Compression therapy: a complete guide. Types of compression bandage. *J Wound Care* **7**(Suppl 2): 5–13

Thomas S, Fram P (2001) The development of a novel technique for predicting the exudate handling properties of modern wound dressings. *J Tissue Viability* **11**(4): 145–60

Thomas S, McCubbin P (2003) A comparison of the antimicrobial effects of four silver-containing dressings on three organisms. *J Wound Care* **12**(3): 101–7

Vowden KR, Vowden P (1999a) Wound debridement, part 1: non-sharp techniques. *J Wound Care* **8**(5): 237–40

Vowden KR, Vowden P (1999b) Wound debridement, part 2: sharp techniques. *J Wound Care* **8**(6): 291–4

Vowden P, Vowden K (2002). Wound Bed Preparation (WBP). *World Wide Wounds.* March. Available: www.worldwidewounds.com/2002/april/Vowden/Wound-Bed-Preparation.html (accessed 17 June 2004)

Index